Advanced Prais

MW00390321

Christina Sell lights the way for yoga teachers and students alike to pay attention to why we do what we do, asking us to consider: *Do we want to be perfect, or do we want to be whole? A Deeper Yoga* offers a quiet contemplation on how we learn to nurture our spirit and create our own mantra of loving kindness for self. With writing prompts and practice suggestions, she invites us to explore the inner deep of our soul. Christina shows us how to use yoga to embrace the self in a blanket of compassion, love and self-respect. This book offers a beautifully written, thoughtful and candid look at how she found peace at last.

— **Michelle Marchildon**, the Yogi Muse,
author of *Fearless After Fifty* and *Finding More on the Mat*

The book is exactly what it promises in its title. It is a deeper yoga to ask such profound questions as, "How might your life shift if you were not consumed with body obsession, food addiction or imposed constructs of improvement?" That question alone is a powerful entry point toward yoga's highest expression, which is freedom through contentment or samādhi. And it reminded me of what I love best about the way Christina writes. Her book is full of similar questions, that can act like keys to unlock every locked door within you. Her path toward a deeper yoga is about making you aware of where you're stuck and giving you the practical tools to get unstuck.

— **Dr. Katy Jane**, Sanskrit & Vedic studies scholar,
meditation instructor & Vedic astrologer;
author of *Awakening with Sanskrit* and *Sanskrit for Yogi*s
www.DrKatyJane.com

Christina Sell is the most effective Hatha Yoga teacher out there, in my experience. She brings that same efficacy to the page. Her written work is not about yoga—it is yoga. This book is an invitation to live the life of yoga, the only life worth living in my world.

— **Darren Rhodes**, author: *Yoga Resource*;
founder, Yogahour; Yogaglo teacher

Christina fearlessly names the dangerous cultural narratives and projections of modern yoga and its insidious harm to the practitioner's psyche and soul when the focus of practice is based solely on outer displays and standards. She invites us toward our own maturation as practitioners, teachers, and imperfect human creatures. We can move beyond the physical practice of yoga and use that same practice as a pathway into deeper intimacy with our thoughts, feelings, behaviors and inner dialogue. Christina's memoir of wholeness through the direct experience of her body and mind illustrates with warmth and honesty what transforms when yoga and psychology work in partnership on one's being. Her book is a must-have for contemporary yoga as we know it now.

— **Livia Cohen-Shapiro**, M.A., Registered Psychotherapist

Reorienting us from our "perfect postures" to an experience of the innermost essence of practice, Christina invites us to "detach from media-driven imperatives" to welcome ourselves to the intimacy we've been seeking since we unrolled a yoga mat for the first time. Reading this evocative work has me returning to my own mat, with my own innate knowing as my finest guide. It will remain near my mat, pages marked and noted, for the rest of my life.

— **Elena Brower**, author: *Practice You and Art of Attention*

Christina Sell, devoted student and respected leader in the field of Yoga, has a well-earned reputation for being a knowledgeable, powerful and life-changing teacher. In A Deeper Yoga she delivers a compelling and inspirational perspective of the transformational power of yoga and skillfully explains how yoga teachers and students can access this depth and then also facilitate others' accessing it for themselves.

— **Desiree Rumbaugh**, Certified Anusara Yoga Instructor and co-author of *Fearless After Fifty: How to Thrive with Grace, Grit and Yoga*

A DEEPER
YOGA

Moving Beyond Body Image
to Wholeness & Freedom

CHRISTINA SELL

HOHM PRESS
Chino Valley, Arizona

© Christina Sell, 2019

All rights reserved. No part of this book may be reproduced in any manner without written permission from the publisher, except in the case of quotes used in critical articles and reviews.

Cover Design: Hohm Press
Interior Design and Layout: Becky Fulker, Kubera Book Design, Prescott, Arizona

Library of Congress Cataloging-in-Publication Data

Names: Sell, Christina, 1969- author.
Title: A deeper yoga : moving beyond body image to wholeness & freedom /
    Christina Sell.
Description: Chino Valley, Arizona : Hohm Press, [2019] | Includes index.
Identifiers: LCCN 2018057175 | ISBN 9781942493457 (trade paperback : alk.
    paper)
Subjects: LCSH: Yoga.
Classification: LCC RA781.67 .S45 2019 | DDC 613.7/046--dc23
LC record available at https://lccn.loc.gov/2018057175

Hohm Press
P.O. Box 4410
Chino Valley, AZ 86323
800-381-2700
http://www.hohmpress.com

This book was printed in the U.S.A. on recycled, acid-free paper using soy ink.

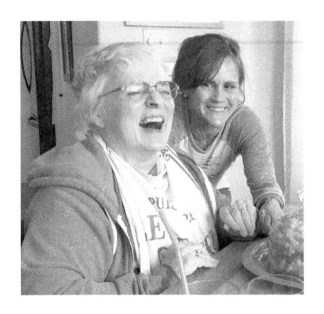

In loving memory of my mother,
Andrea Cheek Frosolono,
with whom I shared the gift of my first breath
and the blessing of her last.

Rest in Peace, Mom.

Andrea Cheek Frosolono
August 8, 1939–February 14, 2018

OTHER BOOKS BY CHRISTINA SELL

Yoga from the Inside Out
Making Peace with Your Body Through Yoga
Hohm Press, 2003

My Body Is a Temple
Yoga as Path to Wholeness
Hohm Press, 2011

CONTENTS

FOREWORD

In the summer of 2014, on a warm evening in the Rocky Mountains of southern Colorado, I found myself engrossed in conversation with Christina Sell. We were in her car in the parking lot of the motel where I was staying during a yoga retreat offered by a well-known Iyengar teacher. Christina too was staying "off campus" and had offered to take me to and from the ranch where the retreat was being held. And so, we rode back and forth together over the course of the six-day intensive.

Sitting in Christina's car each evening after class, we talked and laughed and talked some more. Connecting tentatively at first, we quickly progressed into deep conversation. Be prepared for the same experience as you open *A Deeper Yoga* and read. Her words are honest. They are real. They pierce the pristine veneer of how things are often presented in the yoga world. Christina gets right to the heart of the matter. In these pages, she invites you to do the same. *A Deeper Yoga* is like Christina herself: brave, honest and willing to engage in the occasionally messy process of reflection and introspection. If you allow yourself to be guided by her excellent prompts—for journal writing and personal contemplation—you will find yourself in very unexpected, revealing and enlightened places.

I greatly appreciated our drives together and our parking lot conversations during that Rocky Mountain retreat. We both felt a bit like outsiders at that program. Christina had studied Iyengar yoga for many years but was not a certified teacher in that line, as she was trained in a related yoga tradition. I was a senior-level Iyengar teacher, but one who held an unorthodox approach. We both questioned pretty much everything. And that is what we did, in the car, together. We felt safe in doing so. In your encounter with this book you might feel safe in the same way. Here is a place where you can let your guard down in the company of another. . . a trusted traveler.

On our drives along Highway 160 outside of Durango during that yoga intensive, the conversations traversed a wide variety of topics, yet we talked less about asanas and the various shapes of the poses and more about the bigger picture of how the practice functioned in our lives and relationships. We touched on the many ways in which yoga practitioners give up their personal power and their ability to think critically. We discussed the tendency of many yoga teachers and communities to embrace a kind of group-think, especially the yoga communities that the both of us were brought up in. We acknowledged our own part in all of this, and the complex nature of belonging. We also laid out our struggles with body image, with language, and with our ability or inability to accurately communicate with others about things that are meaningful for us.

The topic of yoga and body image, and concepts of what is or isn't considered beautiful, are covered in depth in this book. Christina shares her personal story of disordered eating, and the pain that it caused her, in a riveting and compelling way. And she manages to bring her excellent sense of humor to all of it.

Christina can be very funny. In fact, I remember us laughing hard together as we recalled one of the retreat teacher's comments about body type. To us, those comments reflected a bias toward a certain type, and we laughed because our similar bodies did not conform to what our teacher apparently preferred. Our mutual laughter was helpful and liberating for me. That teacher's comments could then be considered without heavy emotional reactivity and so provided an opportunity for us to reflect on how *our* words, as teachers, might not support our chosen values in the way that we think they do.

For me, *A Deeper Yoga* feels very much like an ongoing conversation, like the ones I loved having on Highway 160 in which Christina and

Foreword

I questioned everything. We were both giving voice to our questions, feelings and perspectives in a tradition that does not (traditionally anyway) tend to value alternative perspectives. Christina has created space for you, the reader, to join in on the conversation and to speak honestly with yourself from a place of strength and vulnerability. She does this throughout her book in a real way—not presenting a pure and pretty depiction of what some people might feel a female yoga teacher *should* look or sound like. Christina is who she is, as she is, and she writes bravely and truthfully from her heart as well as her gut. These pages are an invitation for you to engage. There space is for you to fill here, and as truthfully as you can.

Christina shares her personal trials and tribulations while keeping a steady eye on the bigger picture. We can do the same. We all experience struggle and connect to each other by sharing these struggles, these stories. As you work with this book you might find yourself surprised—and in a good way—hitting something profound or laughing when you least expect it. Your practice (whether writing or yoga) need not look or sound like anything Christina or anyone else has done: You will be inspired to *follow* her example, not imitate it. It will be your inquiry. It will be your yoga of integration.

—Carrie Owerko, Senior Iyengar Yoga Instructor

INTRODUCTION

———

Recently, after a long hike in the mountains, I went to the local hot springs to soak in the pools. Easing myself slowly into the sublimely hot water, I smiled at the woman on the opposite side of the tub. She smiled back. "I noticed your strength as you walked over here," she said. "What do you do to get that strong? Do you do yoga?"

Feeling a bit awkward, I said, "Well, it's summer so I hike, I bike and I do yoga."

"What kind of yoga?" she asked, adding, "I do yoga. I don't look like you do from yoga."

"It's mostly genetic," I replied.

I soaked in the pool and avoided further eye contact and conversation. However, I continued our dialogue internally, thinking, "Isn't it weird that a woman I have never met felt so free to make a comment about my body?" And secondly, "Isn't it weirder that I felt obligated to answer her?" And thirdly, "With a history like mine, there is simply no easy answer to her question."

Scenes from My Life

Contemplating the question about what I had done to "look like this" evoked flashbacks of my life. Each scene was part of the complicated answer to that seemingly simple inquiry from a stranger.

I am thirteen years old and weigh ninety-eight pounds when my best friend and I go on our first diet. It was called "The Sunshine Diet" and consisted of the same menu for 1-2 weeks: Breakfast: 1 orange, 8 oz. skim milk; Lunch: 1 orange, 8 oz. skim milk, 4 oz. hamburger patty; Dinner: 1 orange, 8 oz. hamburger patty, 8 oz. skim milk. I did lose weight (not that I needed to), but I certainly didn't feel sunny inside.

I am fifteen years old, cheerleading at a football game, when one of the boys in my class yells from the stands, "Nice thunder thighs, Tina." I never enjoyed wearing short skirts much after that moment. In retrospect, it occurs to me that my classmate should have felt ashamed for making a crass, cruel and mean-spirited remark, but instead I was the one who felt embarrassed and belittled.

I am eighteen years old. I am suicidal and a bit strung-out from mixing drugs, alcohol and bulimia. I am talking to my psychiatrist about wanting to get some help. Seizing an opening, she said, "Describe to me what help would look like for you, and I will find it." In that moment of clarity, I laid out, in almost perfect detail, my vision for the treatment center I would enroll in within three months: "I would feel safe enough to be honest about my problems. I would have friends who would not care only about how I looked. I would be able to go swimming and enjoy feeling the water, not just worry about how I showed up in my swimsuit."

I am twenty, and for over three years I weigh and measure my food, according to a protocol of Overeaters Anonymous, in an effort to bring some structure to something as natural as eating, which had become so distorted and out of control that thoughts of suicide enticed me more than once.

More images continued to arise . . . of my healing and recovery work—12-Step groups, psychotherapy, new-age healing circles, a few cults, spiritual communities, schools of yoga and esoteric traditions.

I have tried almost every eating plan imaginable over the last thirty years—raw foods, macrobiotics, low fat/high fiber, South Beach, Atkins, vegan and vegetarian. Each taught me some vital lesson and yet never got close to solving the essential hunger that lived inside me; a hunger for depth, connection and meaning that was insatiable and consuming, and one which no amount of premium ice cream could ever lessen.

I have lived with competing inner injunctions that created a world of double binds—"be skinny" and "don't make anyone else feel uncomfortable by being too thin"; "be disciplined" and "don't be rigid." A move in one direction put love, approval and belonging at stake in a game that could never be won yet demanded I keep playing.

The various milestones of my life have always been marred with the curse of possible weight gain—puberty, freshman year of college, getting married, turning forty, menopause, etc. What a shame that development along the natural arc of life came with the narrative of "don't gain weight, or else," much the way a good legislative bill gets flawed by an oppressive rider, even as it slips through the voting process and gets accepted as law.

A Path of Practice

The dreaded "don't gain weight, or else" has had power over me, my friends and my students and colleagues. Amazing, beautiful, creative and passionate women, who are also kind, smart, hard working and insightful, are often obsessed with how they look. Some of them won't wear bathing suits, others avoid mirrors, and many more exist chiefly on kale smoothies, casting foods like bread or pasta as the enemies.

When I wrote *Yoga From the Inside Out*, a book on yoga and body image in 2003, I thought that yoga would have answers for me and for other women suffering the same or similar thoughts, feelings and behaviors. Thirteen years later, I see overwhelming evidence that yoga may just as likely make matters worse when it comes to body image, weight and food choices.

And yet, that book did prove invaluable for me and for many others as an invitation to ending war with the body while committing to a lifelong peacekeeping effort. It asserted that the truce between society's insane imperatives and one's own inner state could be found only in, and through, a life lived from the heart, dedicated to Grace and grounded in the sanity of sustained practice over time.

With such a long and complicated history involving food and my body, one that would have required a long and complicated answer to the question posed by the stranger in the hot tub about how I got so strong, no wonder I simply deflected the issue, saying, "It's mostly genetics."

Honestly, I have no "5-step Plan for a Strong Body Through Yoga" or a prescribed set of dietary suggestions to offer anyone. I do not actually care what people eat, what kind of exercise they do or even how they look. Nor am I a model of perfection in the areas of food, body image, exercise and health. I prefer breakfast tacos to smoothies; I have stopped trying to overcome my caffeine addiction; and I recognize that no heavy-duty restrictive efforts bear fruit over the long haul . . . for me there is always a swing-back! It may take a week, or it may take a decade, but experience has shown that if I move too far or too fast in any singular direction, the psychic toll necessitates a counterbalance from the other. I have come to appreciate the slow crawl toward change, over and above the grand gestures of seemingly rapid transformation.

In therapy groups I attended in my twenties, there were often older women in the circle. Typically, I was disappointed in them, certain that by the time I was their age I would not have their issues. Surely, all this inner work I was doing in my youth would yield a more "together" older woman. As I am now fifty years old, I see the whole process of change and transformation differently. I no longer value the "perfect picture" on the outside, or the true-but-trite one-liners that attempt to sum up a lifelong process. The deep, honest struggle to *be real now* has my respect . . . along with the humility of repeated efforts and repeated failures. I admire faith, tenacity and any scrap of compassion gained in the work of living a life of meaning, particularly in a body that has weathered the storm of one's own or another's violence. I admire forgiveness. I admire all it takes for any of us to live according to our better angels. (Perhaps I should have shared these things with the woman in the hot tub?)

Why a Deeper Yoga?

If you are holding this book, I assume you have some experience with yoga and some personal history with body image, food addiction, compulsive exercise and/or negative self-esteem. Chances are you have experienced the healing power of postural practice firsthand. You have glimpsed the freedom from stress, the expansion of peace and the awakening of love that so often accompanies breath-based, mindful movement. Perhaps, wanting to share this love with others, you have started teaching. **I wrote this book for you, as an experienced practitioner, and perhaps teacher. While there are plenty of books out there about the benefits of yoga, with great plans for practice and great promises for personal transformation, there are precious few resources to help you when the flush of new love fades, when the practice through which you first experienced self-love has become a source of self-criticism or disillusionment, and/or when the teachers or systems that appeared trustworthy at first, have been exposed as less-than-perfect, misleading, disappointing or perhaps even abusive.** I wrote this book because, if you have struggled with body image, food addiction, compulsive exercise tendencies, and self-criticism, you know how difficult it can be when those issues resurface after any period of respite.

I wrote this book to assure you that hidden in whatever disillusionment, despair or fatigue you may feel about your practice in particular or the industry of yoga in general, you can still find hope and healing through the sustained efforts of practice. I wrote this book to tell you that, while you may have been betrayed, while the practice may seem to create more problems than it solves right now, and while there are horror stories galore about injury, both physical and psychic, chances are that this phase you find yourself in is not a mistake or a result of something going wrong. More likely, this apparent "dark night of the yoga soul" is an invitation to find your own spiritual authority—

to claim your self-compassion at a new, deeper, more empowered level, and to move into a fuller, mature relationship with yourself, your practice and your unique offering in the world.

Reviewing these glimpses of my life, I am amazed that even in the throes of my addictive patterns, a "part" of me *knew exactly* what I needed and even told my psychiatrist what would help me. That wise voice has never left me. And while I have done better and worse jobs of listening to that voice and letting her guidance lead my choices over the years, some essential wisdom was intact back then, even in the midst of a messy life. While this book may not offer a specific plan, I wrote this book to help you get in touch with the wise part of you that is whole, complete and intact, no matter how messy your life currently feels, and to encourage you to trust the guidance that lives within.

Patchwork Quilt

My teacher, Lee Lozowick, called his path "Western Baul." Named after a sect of itinerant beggars in India, the Western version of this Baul path is one of both purity and synthesis. Practice is both formal and ritualized, as well as informal, internal and personal. Lee's teaching was similarly paradoxical—in form he was wildly liberal and staunchly conservative. Trying to pin him down or to summarize the way he taught was often an object lesson in paradox.

The Bauls do not live shut away in caves or holy temples, but sometimes reside in small family ashrams or even on the streets where they perform as traveling minstrels. They declare in overt and subtle ways that the body is a temple and embodiment is a gift. The Bauls sing, dance, perform and practice asana. They are committed to the realization of the Inner Beloved, engaging a blend of *tantric* yoga and *bhakti* yoga that many find offensive and even heretical.

Traditional garb for the Baul consists of patchwork garments constructed of discarded materials. Such a costume exemplifies their commitment to a singular Reality—made whole only by disparate pieces coming together in a unified purpose. Lee's teaching too was a lot like those patchwork jackets—multifaceted and diverse, discarding what no longer worked and creating something new from whatever (or with whomever) was at hand, while simultaneously unified and complete.

My perspectives on yoga and inner work are informed by my own process of synthesis more than as a result of the influence of any one tradition of yoga or any one school of thought. Like a Baul's robe or jacket, this book is a patchwork made from my own experiences and from my continuing efforts to salvage the best of what has been given to me—even what I may have discarded at times—and put it to good use. And, like the Baul musicians who create thousands of songs to the accompaniment of an *ektara*, a one-stringed instrument, I find no better practice in modern times than the one-stringed sadhana of love—our shelter, the focus of all our service, and the aim and expression of all our practice.

This exploration of a deeper yoga has guided my own life trajectory. In the pages that follow, I will share with you some of my failures, successes, weaknesses and strengths . . . and lessons learned. One benefit of spiritual memoir is that a story honestly written can inspire the reader with a more direct and clear understanding of his or her own process. The details of my journey need not match the details of your own. However, my prayer is that, inspired by the general mood of my stories, you will be moved to undertake your unique journey with honesty and clarity. For me, spiritual life involves patching together a quilt of our very own—some synthesis between inner authority and outer structures, between inner validation and outer reflections—all within the dynamic tension of the tradition of yoga and the demands of modern life.

Life will always give us storms to weather. We are in bodies that are both resilient and fragile. If you are alive, then your body is aging, bringing with it yet another set of body-image standards to work with and integrate with compassion and love. In the next year, most of us will get sick, have an injury of some kind, heal, recover, feel exhausted, get rest, gain weight, lose weight, etc. Yoga is not a promise that the ebbs and flows of body-related issues will cease, but is instead a pathway to the inner essence of love wherein wholeness and freedom live.

Cultivating a mood of love is a living commitment to assert, through both attitude and action, that there is a deeper, richer presence embedded into the fabric of life itself. As the commitment deepens within us over time, the context of yoga shifts away from outer ideals to the direct experience that life—and each of us as part of the flow of life itself—with all of its ups and downs is not limited to, defined by or at the mercy of the fluctuations of manifestation. We will be tethered to what is deep within us and the surface-level experiences will be informed by the depths of love. We will realize that *life* has been teaching us all along, and that we are wearing a patchwork jacket of our very own.

PART I

BODY OF LOVE

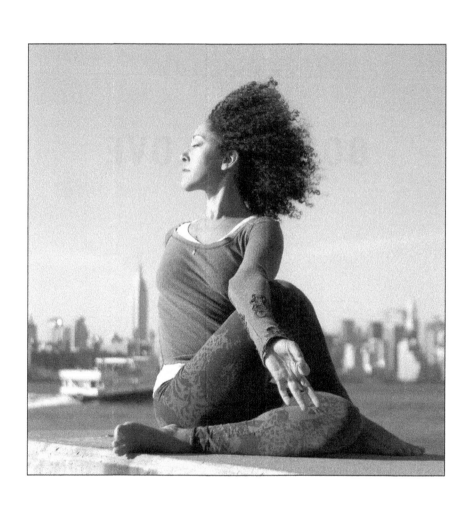

CHAPTER 1

DIVING DEEP & SURFACING

I took my first yoga class in 1991. I don't remember a lot about the class other than how good I felt when class was over. Walking to breakfast after the session, I felt light, free and somehow organized within myself. That feeling of "goodness" became a reference point for a greater possibility than I had ever known in my body.

I was not new to exercise or to stretching or strength-based work. I was a gymnast as a child, a cheerleader as a teen-ager and an aerobics teacher through college. I also was sexually abused as a child, bulimic as a teenager and a compulsive eater and over-exerciser through college. So, while I was not new to exercise, I was new to the sensation of feeling good inside my own body. I began attending yoga classes and practicing some on my own. I developed an intermittent practice along with an interest in Eastern philosophy and personal growth that has continued to develop throughout my life.

These glimpses of goodness make up the essential ingredients in a yoga deeper than image. Over time, these glimpses accumulate and become new reference points of self-understanding, based not on theory or philosophy but on the direct experience of feeling good inside ourselves. The cumulative effect of these experiences, no matter how small or fleeting the glimpses, create the foundation of the transformational process yoga offers.

At War

In 1999, I hit a new low in my relationship to my body. Coming off a relapse cycle of bulimia and compulsive exercise that had taken me into competitive bodybuilding and the extreme dieting seemingly intrinsic to the sport, I had returned to a steady asana practice looking for a way to exercise that would not reinforce my negative thinking and behavioral patterns. I was opened to yoga's possibilities eight years previously, but by '99, asana had devolved for me, becoming more of a background practice: stretching out after a run, or using the postures to recover after a hard week of training. With my descent, returning to yoga felt necessary but also horrible. My muscles were tight and my emotions were frozen from subversion by my compulsive and addictive processes. I lived far from my spirit. The yoga studio where I reengaged the practice seemed full of skinny, happy people who appeared able to enjoy themselves and be "open-hearted" with no problem at all.

To be fair, I had no idea what was going on for anyone in the room because, at the time, I was self-obsessed. I made the classic error in thinking and perception: I compared the way I felt on the inside to how other people looked on the outside. The actual problem I dealt with resided inside my own mind and heart, not in the outer circumstances of the class.

Initially, yoga did not help my body-image issues, nor magically cure my addiction or curb my compulsions. Even though everyone did their best to be welcoming and inclusive, I felt alone. Even though nobody said a word about appearance, I remained focused on how I looked. Even though no one hinted at competition, I could not stop comparing myself to others. And while my teacher was saying things like "make your pose an offering" and "express the posture from the beauty of your heart," all I felt was stiff, tight and angry. And sad. In fact, as the teacher's relentlessly-affirming instructions continued, I felt worse, not better.

Yoga did not seem to help me . . . at least not right away.

And, yoga did allow me to see myself clearly in the moment. I became acutely aware of how alienated I felt from myself and how violent I had been to myself over the years. I knew with stark, painful clarity that I could not go on hating my body and punishing myself through exercise, diets and negative self-talk. I knew I had been at war with my body. I also knew my only option was to find a way to make peace.

Initial Steps in Peacemaking

I wrote *Yoga from the Inside Out: Making Peace with Your Body Through Yoga* in 2001 as a way to articulate and integrate my peacemaking process. In the book, published in 2003, I discussed and told stories about the healing power of yoga. I also pointed to the insidious nature of modern society's values, which I called "the Sleeping World," within the yoga industry, arguing the dysfunctional cultural norms for beauty were nested in our perceived spiritual separation:

> The Sleeping World functions according to laws of separation, competition, judgment, domination, submission and division. In terms of body image and self-esteem, the Sleeping World holds us hostage to ideals for the human body that are unrealistic, often unhealthy, and founded on a lack of respect for our essential worthiness and goodness.[1]

In this same book, I asserted practitioners could either engage yoga in a way that reinforced the values of the Sleeping World, or practice in a way to loosen the knot of separation and expose the myth of suffering. I described the transformational power of intention and attention.

---

[1]   Christina Sell, *Yoga from the Inside Out*, Chino Valley, Arizona: Hohm Press, 2003, 18.

5

I explored how directly experiencing oneself as a multifaceted being
would loosen the hold of the Sleeping World's cultural imperatives
and provide an enlarged reference point for identity, well-being and
embodiment. Pictures of two-dozen white and black women, each
joyfully practicing yoga postures, graced the book. These women,
who were not professional models, had bodies that did not conform
to the images of beauty portrayed in the yoga magazines and other
publications of the time.

While the book was well received, many students and other
readers asked questions and made comments such as, "How can I
actually do what you are talking about?" and "I know you say to make
yoga a peace offering, but no one ever talks about that in my classes."
I realized my failure to adequately communicate the concept that
the requisite work was essentially an inside job, one in which healing
negative body image and its manifestations were inextricably linked
to spiritual practice and to one's maturity as a practitioner.

In 2008, I began another manuscript, this one titled *My Body Is
a Temple: Yoga as a Path to Wholeness,* which was published in 2011.
This time, I applied the principles originally outlined in *Yoga from the
Inside Out* to yoga practice *beyond* asana. I encouraged practitioners to
expand their understanding of the body over and above the limits of
their physicality, and suggested ways to develop a body of practice, a
body of knowledge, and a body of experience through yoga principles
and practice.

Here again, I urged readers to look within themselves to determine
what is needed for a personal, authentic, sane and life affirming
relationship with yoga. I made distinctions between the practice of
yoga and the yoga industry, and between yoga class and personal time
on the mat alone. I invited everyone to consider how best to bring
the principles of yoga philosophy to life in their daily circumstances
without rigidity or dogma.

Where Are We Now?

I am writing this book in 2018, seventeen years after I wrote *Yoga from the Inside Out* and ten years after I wrote *My Body Is a Temple*. I have taught yoga classes, workshops and training sessions for over twenty years. Reflecting on the diverse trends in the world of yoga I witnessed over these years—the birth of Facebook, Twitter, Instagram, YouTube, online classes, blogs, vlogs and podcasts—I am not surprised to see the flowering of the seeds of dysfunction I identified so many years ago. With more people practicing some form of yoga, and with the enormous economic impact of such widespread participation, the values of the Sleeping World obviously have infiltrated the world of yoga, much in the way I predicted and warned about in 2003. This infiltration uses the power of slick marketing to create high expectations about what yoga can do, while promising success, beauty and well-being according to the Sleeping World's standards. Through the mechanisms of social media, anyone can now easily participate in the proliferation of images reinforcing the values of a sick, societal norm.

In 2003, two primary industry magazines and a handful of books and VHS videos were available for the general public. Those resources pictured lithe, young and bendable yoga practitioners and set up a "yogic ideal" of beauty no different from conventional society's standards. These "model" practitioners were also seasoned teachers, dedicated students and sincere devotees. The problem was not that they were featured in these publications, but that other highly accomplished, yet less-conventionally beautiful practitioners were never included. In effect, then, the Sleeping World's standards determined who was the expert and who wasn't. Instead of yoga creating a countercultural environment, the yoga industry indoctrinated us more deeply with the cultural values of the Sleeping World.

Notably, however, out of the current social-media cacophony, other important trends have emerged—trends that encourage a more positive body orientation in yoga. By consciously using the channels of social media and publishing, various social movements are working to expand the ideals of beauty beyond conventional society's "thin ideal," and are tirelessly aiming to create a more inclusive and affirming atmosphere for yoga practice and personal expression.

I am inspired to see how the work I began in 2001 has developed in mainstream yoga culture. We can now find images of practitioners of all sizes and shapes in workshop brochures, training manuals, books, calendars and ads for apparel. (For recommendations about this mounting body of work, please see the Resources section at the back of the book.)

Still, such inclusion is insufficient. Personally, I want the work of yoga to continue beyond diverse ad campaigns and products aimed at validating and accommodating the ever-expanding demographic of modern-day yoga practitioners. As important as those outcomes are, yoga practice can orient us *beyond* culture, image and beauty—not simply improve or elevate the narrative of those domains.

The work of a deeper yoga will not be easy or immediate. But, orienting our lives internally and according to essential and chosen values, rather than by conditioned injunctions, will connect us to our inner wisdom and free us from dependency on outside sources of validation and approval.

Transformation Is Ongoing

The transformational path requires progress not perfection; perseverance and patience rather than gratification and easy answers. Each of us lives in an always changing body in a network of always changing relationships and in an always changing culture. Within these fields of change, yoga practice directs us to find a connection to what is unchanging within us, our innermost Self. Nonetheless, even were we to find and experience the big "It"—the changeless Reality within us—no place at which we arrive and "finish up" exists. There is simply the unrelenting flow of life, with no real conclusion in sight. We must still go on living on Planet Earth, in our current culture, in a complex web of relationships, in a body that ages and dies, cycling though periods of health and sickness. Whatever we encounter, we have to just keep going.

> A master of a specific form of Japanese dance was asked about the necessity of practice. He replied, "Once you have mastery, it is then that you can truly practice. Even when mastery is attained you must keep going. In fact, all you ever really have is "keep going."

Writing this book has been like pulling over to the side of the road in my journey of "Keep Going," giving me an opportunity to reflect and share about both my own personal process and the unfolding culture of modern yoga. Although my understanding has matured over the years, and the nature of the yoga industry has shifted as well, essentially, the work of making peace with the body, of practicing a yoga of wholeness, of moving beyond image and into direct knowledge and freedom, is the same as it ever was. There is the repeated task of meeting the moment as it is, embracing it fully and surrendering to it as a gesture of reverence, devotion and intention in action. Practices, techniques and protocols are endless, and yet they all point inward—to what lives deeper than and underneath the vicissitudes of the body, mind and emotions. All yogic practice invites us to bring our inner recognition into our ordinary waking lives with increasing degrees of integrity and congruence.

From the moment we wake up in the morning, our senses draw us into the world that we see, taste, touch, smell and hear in a continual attempt to orient our external reference point and identity. Culture, society and personality all reinforce this external orientation and identification in both pleasurable and painful manifestations. The gift of yoga practice and yoga-inspired technology resides not in the denial of the outer world and its pleasure and pain, but in the re-orientation of our reference points to our internal field of energy. The re-orientation involves a process and a life's work, not a quick fix or a magic formula. Essentially, the transformational process asks us to take a hero's journey, away from the familiar landmarks of our conditioning and into the wilderness of our inner landscape.

The Work of Transformation

If we stay true to the course of personal growth, we will cross many thresholds. In the crossing, we become no longer the person we knew ourselves to be, and yet we may not know for sure who or what we are becoming. Personally, I am most interested in this in-between stage of the process, even though doubt, worry, insecurities and fear accompany the "threshold passage." When we no longer have a grasp on the things we have always known to be true—about ourselves, each other, the world, etc.—we are the most vulnerable to the many voices of fear, such as: *What if it is always like this? Maybe I never should have walked through the gateway of this change. Maybe there is nothing on the other side. Who am I if I am not what I was? Who will I be? What if I don't like it?*

Our identity structures—our patterns of thought and behavior—will be the very material that makes our transformational passage possible. As the gestation process takes time, it will follow its own intelligent pace. We will not jump through the threshold, moving from one way of seeing and functioning to another through an all-at-once event.

Intellectually, we may know transformation means we must be "undone" in some way to be "born again." Yet we can easily forget that such a process, by its very nature, involves difficulties and pain—"undone" represents a type of dismemberment. We may forget that a sense of being "dis-membered" is not a bad thing, a sign that the process is not working, or an indication that the yoga has become ineffective. In fact, I believe quite the opposite. While we may have stepped onto the path to "feel better," the cost for feeling better is often feeling worse for a period of time.

Without an honest experience of one's own suffering, transformation will remain elusive. The struggle with body image, for example, will not be overcome by referencing a persona with perfect self-love and unrelenting and positive self-esteem. The pain of the struggle itself will be what creates the longing to move beyond the constraints in which we find ourselves. The desire for a connection to what is more real than self-obsession and self-concern will emerge, not from our perfection, but from our suffering and resultant humility.

We will evolve in, through and beyond the structures that have defined us. As our deepest soul's instincts clarify and emerge, the longing of our heart will create a connection to our spiritual source. Then, we can access what will sustain and inform us throughout the destruction of our old ideas of who we are and allow us to live from our enlarged reference points.

To be clear, I do not think we always need: to feel worse in order to grow, to believe in suffering unnecessarily in the name of spiritual growth and transformation, or to martyr ourselves or accept abuse, shame and/or humiliation from our inner critics, outer teachers and/or communities. I am talking here about an inner state of discomfort that, while rarely pleasant, carries within it an imprint of deep psychic change, of a truth of the heart calling us to come into integrity with who we most truly are. In view of my own experience, this state carries an exquisite flavor of something real, deeply nourishing and simultaneously humbling. Decidedly different from complaining, victimhood or blaming, the discomfort I am speaking of feels "right" to my spirit, even if it feels "wrong" to some aspect of my thinking mind.

Whenever I have walked through a certain kind of change or empowering shift, the walking through, the leap of faith, and the process itself was the teacher and the agent of the shift or change. If, for instance, the process was never scary, how would we learn the depth of our courage? If we were never at risk of being betrayed, how would we understand trust? We cannot, for instance, learn patience quickly. We cultivate faith in the face of fear, confidence in the face of doubt and compassion in the midst of one another's and our own suffering.

Beyond Competence

My therapist once cautioned me about making life too much about competence and doing things right. Life, with its many complexities, features paradox, mistake-making, triumphant achievement and abysmal failure. We love, hate, betray, forgive and continue on. I was reminded of my therapist's caution in the hours after my mother passed, when the issue of a "good death" came up around the dinner table.

My mom spent the last six days of her life in the hospital before dying from complications of pneumonia. Her breathing was labored, she seemed confused, and letting go was not easy. I had my hand on her heart as she exhaled for the final time. Sharing the confusion, the struggle, the fear and the final breath with her was an experience that lived in a world beyond right and wrong, good and bad. How ludicrous to assign a "good" or "bad" label to something so mysteriously natural as death. And, by the same token, how unfair to judge our living, breathing moments by the limiting narrative of competence and skill, or good and bad.

What Do You Reach For?

My spiritual teacher once said we can know the state of our spiritual practice by observing where we turn when we are in crisis. Do we run to old patterns or do we turn to something higher and deeper? Do we take refuge in fear and patterned behaviors or do we seek refuge in the company of seekers? Do we look to society to validate our inner life or do we take refuge in the truth of our hearts and the wisdom of the teachings we study and practice? Learning to reach beyond our patterns during the passage through our transformational thresholds defines what a life of practice is about. No matter how sincere, ardent or hardworking we may be, each of us will fall down, fail in our efforts and forget our aim. Repeatedly.

The good news is that the path of wholeness does not reflect some kind of all-or-nothing game where getting it "right" once and for all constitutes success. Much of the work lives in knowing what to reach for, and how to reach for it when we are down. I see this work as a continual re-orienting away from false beliefs into the direct experience of the field of love within. Re-orienting does not require a perfect diet, advanced yoga postures, fame, fortune or trendy clothes. Re-orienting ourselves happens in the midst of the nitty-gritty details of our lives and in the sometimes-messy world of relationships.

Writing to the Depths

Throughout this book you will find suggestions for practice, and writing assignments aimed at helping you use my ideas and perspectives as springboards to dive into your own inner work. Writing provides a means by which *you* can listen to *you*—to your inner wisdom, your truth and your perspectives. Writing gives us an opportunity to articulate our experiences as accurately and honestly as possible. Over time, this practice helps us learn to validate our own wisdom and deepen our capacity for self-trust. Without the capacity for self-validation and integration, the many well-intended yogic practices will tend to create self-judgment, self-doubt and self-criticism as opposed to self-empowerment, clarity and trust. Writing can help you:

- listen to your own inner wisdom
- reflect on your personal experience
- gain insight, self-knowledge and self-expression
- integrate experience into living and embodied wisdom

And, perhaps most importantly, writing can be whatever else you need it to be for your growth. In Chapter 8, I will explore this subject of writing in greater detail. Feel free to turn there now or at anytime you need encouragement in the practice.

Preparation for Writing

1. **Write by hand.** Of course you are free to use your laptop for writing practice. But, in my experience, there is a more direct connection between the pen in the hand and the heart. Writing by hand encourages me to gently consider and carefully entrust each word to the paper. Or, it allows me to simply scribble and cross things out, and not delete them right away, just for the reminding mess of it!
2. **Choose a notebook that makes you happy.** The size, shape, line spacing and texture of paper in a notebook will make a difference in encouraging (or discouraging) you in your writing practice. Find one that you feel comfortable and beautiful with. You'll want to carry it around to a café or a sacred space sometimes, and the notebook should reflect your commitment to yourself and your life.
3. **Choose a pen that works well for you.** While some folks like to write in pencil or colored marker, these media can sometimes discourage a type of serious reflection as you write. Pencil will fade. Colored markers might bleed through to the other side of your paper. A pen is matter of personal preference. Be discriminating.
4. **Write only for yourself.** This is easier said than done, but definitely worth the challenge. As you write, become aware of "who" or "what" you are trying to please or impress or convince. When you notice this, shift your intention and

then keep writing with this awareness. Gently observe what happens. Write about what you are discovering.

5. **Sometimes write with a friend.** Some of us find it hard to carve out time to write. If you have a trusted friend, or fellow yoga student who seems willing, invite them to join you in a writing date. Keep the session short, like 10-15 minutes of writing, followed by tea and conversation. Share your writing only if you wish.

6. **Date and Topic.** Date your work and start each new assignment on a clean notebook or journal page. Write out the question or topic you are responding to at the top of the page. Years from now you will be happy to have this record of your progress both in self-understanding and in your ease with writing.

7. **Go with the Muse.** As you start to address one writing prompt or one question, you may find you are suddenly swept into a completely different subject with much more creative juice for you in the moment. Trust this! Nobody else cares. It's your call. Follow where the energy leads you. If you find yourself blocked, not knowing where to turn next, simply start over on a clean page. Or, write: "What I'm really trying to say is…" and continue. Have fun. Maybe a story will evolve. Maybe a poem will emerge. Don't stop it.

Writing Prompts to Start With

Choose one of the following and spend 10-15 minutes writing about it. Then, take another prompt and write some more. Enjoy.

1. In what ways has yoga helped you to bring your attention inward?

2. In what ways do you find it difficult to let go of outside imperatives, expectations and assumptions? Consider your life both "on" and "off" your mat.

3. How do you relate to the concepts of competence and "good and bad" when it comes to yoga practice and study?

4. What might shift in your life if you were free of concepts like "good and bad" and lived from wholeness and acceptance instead?

5. Based on the material covered in the Introduction, reflect and write: If your spiritual life was a patchwork jacket, what are some of the pieces you have sewn together? What pieces of fabric have you discarded? Why?

Once again, freedom and peace do not live in achieving or conforming to outer standards but in the recognition and experience of our inner wholeness. When we glimpse the fullness of who we are, we find that love is our true nature. New possibilities show up because we have created a new reference point for our relationship to ourselves, to our bodies and to our life of spiritual practice.

—Christina Sell

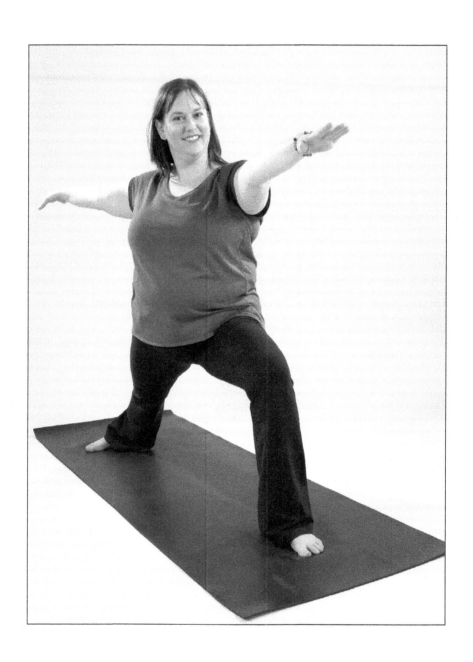

CHAPTER 2

BEYOND BODY IMAGE

———————

There are two primary pathways in yoga. The first pathway of energy is an inward-moving flow toward the heart of who we are. This path often travels through the painful territory of our past wounds, future fears, current frailties and the various defense mechanisms we have erected in an attempt to safeguard what is most precious within us. Underneath this myriad of conditioned patterns lives our essential nature, free from the constraints of the past and the fears for the future, radiating what sacred traditions often refer to as the "light of the soul."

The second pathway is an outgoing flow of energy, an authentic expression of the knowledge gained from the inward journey. Modern life and most self-help strategies are primarily aimed at improving the outward-flowing stream of energy. We set goals, we make lists, we clean up our eating, we lose weight, we get a better job, we attain challenging yoga postures, we manage our time better. In short, we improve ourselves. On the societal level, the outward-flowing stream manifests in various forms of activism in which we diligently work to create more just, equitable and sane expressions of humanity. We support fair legislation; we work for policy changes that address and seek to rectify the imbalances of power, privilege and opportunity.

All of this outer work can be helpful, and yet, mounting evidence suggests legislation does not solve the problems of racism, sexism and our collective, deep-rooted cultural prejudices, just as diets rarely result in lasting weight loss or freedom from the obsession with food and appearance. When we primarily work with the outer stream of our life circumstances, either personally or collectively, we run the risk of our efforts and changes being largely cosmetic. If we only tend to the inner, we run the risk of being myopic, self-centered and even somewhat narcissistic. When we do not know ourselves well, and/or when that knowledge cannot find optimal, creative expression, we will be at war with ourselves and with one another. When these two pathways of energy come together—when the inner knowledge of our deepest self finds authentic expression in our behavior—we have integrity and peace. We live an outer life congruent with our inner life.

For yoga to move deeper than image, we need to use the techniques of asana, breath-work, chanting and visualization to facilitate an inward understanding, as well as to promote an authentic outer expression. Asana practitioners often have difficulty using the shapes and positions of the body to go inward, because so much time and attention is spent on the exterior form of the poses and how to execute them. The source of our suffering lives on the outer or superficial level of asana when we compare the shapes our body can make to those of others pictured in books, magazines or Instagram feeds.

Or, perhaps we expect to be as compassionate, loving and selfless as the saints and sages of the stories and scriptures were said to be. Meanwhile, our messy, complicated humanity is pitted against our deep, spiritual longing—becoming proof, once again, that we are flawed, imperfect and unworthy.

No one can live for long on the surface with all of its competing imperatives without getting beaten up and burned out. Too much time in comparison, judgment and chasing outside standards of success will compromise our capacity to live in the sense of wonder we might have initially found in yoga. We must move down deeper, away from images, rules and unrealistic expectations, even if our surface efforts have been well intentioned. That is, even if we *really want* to be "good yogis."

Hidden in every shape, every alignment cue, every "do this" and "don't do this" is a call to pay attention: first to the shape, then to the placement of our body, then to the actions that activate the posture, then to the effects on our body, mind and mood, and finally to the part of us that watches it all. Alignment in yoga is far from an exhaustive list of perfection-oriented details, but is, instead, a call to pay attention to who we are at increasingly deep and more subtle layers of our being. The shapes are not there to fuel self-criticism, self-judgment or self-obsession. We do not need to be thin, fit, strong or look like a magazine model to start the process of paying attention to placement, action and the effect they have on our consciousness. Not one thing on the surface must be perfect or handled completely before we can go inward toward our source.

The work of re-orienting ourselves toward interior values is the primary aim of this book. This book is not an exhaustive treatise on yoga, is not a great beginner's manual and will make no recommendations about food, diet or weight-loss. Instead, this book intends to provide inspiration and encouragement to go deeper into your own conditioned beliefs and behaviors so that you can glimpse a freedom sourced inside yourself, rather than being dependent on outside approval and validation.

Image and Experience

I first heard the term "body image issues" in the 1980s in association with eating-disorder education. With anorexia and bulimia on the rise, body dysmorphia was entering the mainstream discussion. Thousands of young women whose body weight fell into healthy, normal ranges were looking in mirrors and seeing themselves as fat, unacceptable and in need of a body overhaul. I was one of these young women.

Nowadays, I hear the words "body image" to refer to a more general self-hating malaise people have about their bodies, and the ways that their body falls short of cultural ideals. As a society, we have lost our ability (assuming we ever had the ability in the first place) to maintain a perspective on the insanity that marketing agencies everywhere are selling, in an effort to make us feel so terrible about who we are that our only obvious option for salvation will be to buy their products. And the noise of this particular narrative has become so loud that it is almost impossible to bear up against it.

Not only marketing agencies drive body dissatisfaction. Fat shaming and fat discrimination cost many people jobs, promotions and pay raises. Conscious and unconscious racial biases determine outcomes for people based solely on the color of their skin, creating a thicket of problems from self-esteem and internalized shame, to limited opportunities for education, jobs and housing, to poverty and even to violence. Racial oppression is inextricably linked to the body, as the history of slavery shows the outrageous reality of owning other people's bodies and controlling them for personal gain. Gender bias and sexual orientation create yet another labyrinth of discriminatory issues to cope with, as people struggle to reconcile the experience of who they are, with the body they have, within a culture that only recognizes a small range of acceptable possibilities. In our youth-obsessed culture, aging offers most people new challenges to face, where the inevitable changes in one's appearance trigger doubt, insecurity and feelings of invisibility. And, negative body image is like the multi-headed Hydra of Greek mythology—as soon as you cut off one head of this creature, two more sprout in its place. Society's imperatives of oppression are relentless, multifaceted and pervasive.

A mounting body of work—written for both scholarly and public audiences, from both academic and personal perspectives—outlines and catalogues the many decapitated heads of the negative-body-image beast I am describing. The many heads share a similar root—the assumption of separation from our spiritual source and our energetic interconnectedness. This assumed separation keeps us identified with our bodies and our thoughts and with shallow, culturally-defined imperatives. My interest as a yoga practitioner and teacher looks to this root for a solution, much in the way that the Hydra in Greek mythology was ultimately defeated. In the myth, the hero Heracles decapitated each head and then cauterized the stump, preventing any future heads from growing.

Yoga philosophy and practice offers us helpful technology for working directly with our thoughts, feelings, perceptions and sensations in ways that can shift our orientation away from the outer world and toward our inner, spiritual source. The solution for negative body image will be found when we reference our worth in something deeper than the body, and when we dismantle the power of our conditioned mind so that we can see the reality of who we are more clearly. Recognizing our spiritual essence is the means through which we can cauterize the wound of our culture and psychology, and prevent the growth of continued and painful manifestations. Whereas the outward moving stream is often more communal, where we take action to improve our shared world, the inward moving path of this work is highly personal. It requires us to move through our own biographical history with clarity and courage.

Emotional/Spiritual Implications of Asana

While asana clearly uses the physical body for practice, asana can also be a tool for self-knowledge and spiritual insight. Asana offers much more than a physical practice. Asana incorporates the invitation to *be inside* the body through observation, sensation and direct perception. The efficacy of asana to heal the root causes of our body-image issues results from the way practitioners can use the poses to direct their attention inward—beyond the boundaries of the body and beyond concerns with image and appearance. Glimpsing the inner aspects of one's being in asana, we then have an opportunity to re-orient ourselves away from *image and ideal*, and toward a larger sphere of self-understanding. When the larger sphere of self-understanding becomes our *direct experience*, body image issues become re-contextualized and our yoga drops deeper. We may still wish we were thinner or different-looking, but from our new vantage point we might also see those wishes and thoughts as less convincing and less meaningful. Old patterns of thought, feeling and behavior may still arise as habits, but they can lose their obsessive or compulsive hold on us. In this way, nothing changes ... and everything changes.

No easy path exists through this re-contextualizing, peacemaking process. Like most things in yoga, sustained efforts over a long period of time are required for the work to take root inside of us and bear fruit. As sincere as we may be about wanting to shift our relationship to body image through yoga, our habits of negative self-talk and shame-based criticism commonly come to the forefront and discourage, if not drown out, an attempt to be breath-focused, attentive to alignment, or aware of ourselves energetically and spiritually.

Unfortunately, our negative thoughts do not arrive waving a flag of warning to tell us, "For the next sixty minutes, I am going to give you a run for your money to see if you really can break free of your patterns and conditioning like you say you want to. Get ready. It is going to be rough, but you can do it." Instead, self-hatred and self-criticism—be they the internalized messages of childhood, culture or both—come in riding our emotions. We then easily feel ashamed, ugly, unlovable, different and bad. Like a toxic miasma of self-loathing, these messages come to us from inside our own emotional body and increase the difficulty of gaining clarity and perspective. *What is happening?* we wonder. *Why do I feel so bad?* we ask, and *What can I do about the situation I find myself in?*

In my experience, too many people come to yoga classes or to their mats looking for a break from their inner demons, only to find the "enemy" has rolled out its own mat inside their emotional body and inside their head. Consumed by negative self-talk and the shame-based feelings I am describing, many practitioners commonly feel that yoga, the class and/or our teacher have somehow betrayed us.

A Peaceful Revolution

Fifteen years ago, I thought yoga had a magical power to bring about transformation with respect to body image. I now see yoga as a tool, not an answer or a solution in and of itself. In the same way that a hammer can be used to build a temple of great beauty, that identical tool can damage, destroy and cause harm. From my observations, a person is just as likely to feel worse about his or her body as a result of practicing yoga than they are to feel better.

As discussed in Chapter 1, I also believe the seeds of transformation are planted in that moment of "feeling worse" and that, in those moments when shame has us in its grip, or when comparison is tormenting us, we are crossing a threshold on our path of healing. If, when faced with the many ways we might be "feeling worse," we can turn our attention to our breath, to an action of alignment, to the direct experience of sensation in our body as we hold a pose or flow through a *vinyasa*, or to the remembrance of our Spiritual Heart, I believe we can slowly, over a long period of time, keep walking along the path of the inward moving stream, do the work of disarming the Sleeping World's imperatives inside of us and move toward our inner wisdom.

Yoga as a Personal Practice

When I say "yoga," I refer to a combination of yoga-inspired technologies, psychological tools, spiritual perspectives and practices that help re-orient us from the outer body—from image and self-obsession—to the direct experience of our inner essence. I believe that the best chance for using yoga as a healing technology resides in personal practice. Internal focus can be maximized and practitioners can tailor practice to their specific needs. For me, classes and workshops function best as adjuncts for personal practice, rather than as the primary access to self-understanding. A group can actually be a distracting influence: Any group dynamic challenges us to sort through a variety of opinions and influences. Once we are better established in self-knowing through personal practice, navigating the terrain of ongoing public classes may be easier and less demanding.

I am not saying that attending public classes and workshops is wrong. Quite the opposite. Because the solitary world of personal practice can be very difficult, group instruction may be very useful at many points along the way. Nonetheless, many of the concepts and skills vital to shifting perspective about oneself need to be explored *internally* and thereby made personal. These concepts and skills are profoundly empowering when implemented independently, in contrast to expecting or requiring someone else to facilitate an essentially individual process.

When I began practicing asana in 1991, my teacher offered two beginning-level classes each week. I went to class regularly and enjoyed them greatly. After a few weeks, I asked my teacher how I could do yoga more often. I expected her to tell me to come to her intermediate-level classes. Instead, she recommended two books and told me I should practice at home on the days when the beginner's class did not meet. I took her advice and set up a personal practice schedule. My asana practice has always been a predominantly private and personal endeavor. I have rarely gone to class daily and have always done the bulk of my studies with my teachers through books, workshops and occasional classes.

As asana has increased in popularity, I have seen several changes in the landscape of asana instruction and practice. With more people making a living as yoga teachers and more studios serving the growing interest in the practice of asana, the majority of practitioners and teachers rely on public classes for practice. In the average metropolitan area, there may be a yoga studio in every neighborhood, and a host of classes to choose from every hour. I am sure that, if I had started yoga in the current milieu, I would never have stabilized such a personal practice because I would not have needed to. When I began there were two classes I was allowed to attend. If I wanted to do yoga on a daily basis, I was responsible for establishing a practice.

The commerce of the situation is clear—studios and teachers rely on daily participation in classes for the revenue that allows staying in business. And while the business model is perfectly understandable, many of the resultant dynamics are troubling, and even counterproductive for untangling the knots of our conditioning that keep us identified with external sources for validation of our self-worth.

Classes are wonderful places for providing community, connection, education and inspiration. For many people, a group setting is vital for experiencing this healing power of community. A bond forms among people who practice together regularly—people who bear witness to the ups and downs of one another's lives both on and off the yoga mat. And, personal practice is important for developing autonomy, independence, self-reliance and self-empowerment. In my view, the best chance we have for using yoga to help us detach from culturally-determined and media-driven imperatives lives in the optimal balance between personal practice and public classes. Simply put, I do not think a yoga class embedded in the consumer-driven culture is likely to produce freedom from that culture.

Too often when yoga practitioners hear about personal practice, they feel ashamed that they do not practice alone. It is as though everyone "knows" they should practice at home but they don't, for various reasons. Once shame is triggered, defensiveness often follows, which gets projected onto whatever authority seems to be preaching about personal practice at the time. Or the shame becomes self-hatred and, instead of being projected outward, is internalized and directed inward. I don't wish to participate in that dynamic. Many troubling aspects of modern yoga culture—finances, affordability, accessibility, and the inevitable comparisons of ability, size, shape, flexibility and strength that occur where two or more are gathered—go away in the privacy of one's personal practice. A personal practice can be tailor made to meet your specific needs, and provides a way to enter directly into a personal, specific, respectful and kind friendship with yourself. Of course, the relationship with oneself in personal practice resembles any other relationship in life—intimacy takes time to develop, and the pathway there is often boring and ordinary.

I do not expect anyone to jump suddenly from going to public classes *only*, to having a personal practice *only*. Nor do I expect asana practitioners to suddenly embrace and enjoy meditation or pranayama. If you love your ongoing public classes, I think you should keep going. If asana is your primary yogic technology, keep practicing! The distinction I am making between public class and personal practice is not an either/or, but simply an explanation of the context I hold about body image, freedom and wholeness. By all means, go to classes and do "the work" there as you can. And, as you are ready, *if you are ready*, slowly introduce a solitary, personally-guided practice into your life.

Personal Work, Group Setting

Eventually, distinctions between personal practice and group instruction will blur. Over time, a mature practitioner grows to understand they put themselves in a group setting for the opportunity to do personal work. While it appears that we pay money for a class or a workshop so that the teacher will give us information, or talk us through a routine, in actuality we are paying for the opportunity to work on ourselves in a group setting. We pay not to be shielded from comparison, but to confront the pattern of comparison and move through it. We pay not to be guided through a practice, but to learn the skills to guide ourselves through. We pay not for everything to be made easier, but to have an opportunity to grow our capacity to meet challenges, whether those challenges are physical, emotional, intellectual or spiritual.

From a more esoteric perspective, even when practicing alone, we have the energetic support and company of our teachers and community behind our efforts. Even when I am alone on my mat, I draw upon the wellspring of knowledge my teachers have shared with me over the years to guide my efforts.

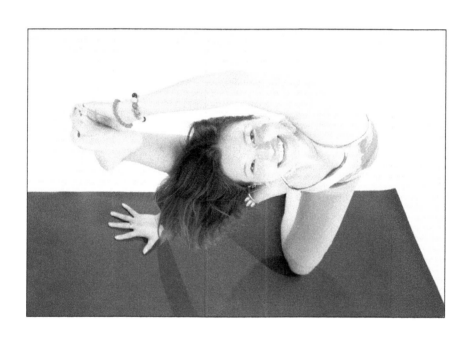

CHAPTER 3

HEALING PERFECTIONISM

Yoga allows you to rediscover a sense of wholeness in your life.
—B.K.S. Iyengar

Yoga is the state of missing nothing.
—Sri Brahmananda Saraswati

The Sanskrit word *purna* means "fullness," "wholeness" and the "perfect." According to this definition, something is perfect at its fullness; when it is whole. Accordingly, a perfect person is a whole person; a perfect pose is performed completely, when the fullness of the body's current capacity joins with the fullness of mindful attention; a perfect body is *complete* with both the limits and potentials of its physicality.

By contrast, modern culture generally considers something perfect when it is without flaw or absent of fault. According to this paradigm, a perfect pose looks like the picture in the book; a perfect person has no flaws or faults, and a perfect body looks like that of one of the airbrushed models in magazines.

Of course, the operative cultural definition gets tricky because the notion of "no flaw" or "no fault" immediately begs the question—"according to what standard?" For instance, following a diet *perfectly* depends on which diet you are talking about. Eating meat is essential on the Atkins diet, but eating meat on a vegetarian diet constitutes failure. Being round and voluptuous gave Marilyn Monroe a perfect body in her era, but perfection in the 1960s required Twiggy's skinnier proportions. Being perfect in modern life is always in reference to an outer standard. And, more often than not, that outer standard is determined according to a set of oppressive biases regarding race, gender, physical ability and appearance.

Herein lies the problem of using outer standards to define and assess ourselves: We will be consciously, or unconsciously, linking our value and worth to a standard that is ever-changeable, conventionally-determined, essentially arbitrary and fundamentally oppressive. Even if we meet the outer standard perfectly, which is extremely doubtful, who is to say that the reference point for that perfection won't shift with the next marketing trend, or that the standard we are conforming to has any alignment with our best interests?

> Perfectionism is a toxic belief that often feeds dysfunctional thinking, feeling and behavior. Making peace with the body is not about whipping ourselves into shape, cleaning up our diets, or suddenly loving ourselves exactly as we are. Instead, peace begins when we meet ourselves as we are, acknowledge our suffering, and find more compassion for ourselves, our struggles, and what we perceive to be our shortcomings.
>
> —Christina Sell

For many, this unexamined notion of perfection produces considerable psychological misery. For example, most families have both consciously-stated and unconsciously-determined standards for perfection. Meet the standards, you are loved. Fall short of the standards, love is revoked. Commonly, the threat of love being revoked colors the family's psychic atmosphere and leads to psychological instability and anxious uncertainty. Also, within the family dynamic, these standards of perfection create and influence a whole range of "acceptable" beliefs along with expectations for children: Expectations about their physical appearance, behavior, temperament and personality. Acceptable beliefs about race, gender, politics and religion…and more. Falling short of the ideals—a mixture of culturally-, societally- and familially-conditioned patterns—results in "losing" love or being "cast out" in some way. To further complicate issues, for various reasons many children *feel* "cast out," even with parents who love them deeply.

We see the same acceptance-rejection patterns in many religious or spiritual communities as well. Religions often require perfect compliance with the outer structures of their rules and regulations as the entry fee for belonging, being loved and/or being saved. Having faults and flaws in a highly-dogmatic religious community can have tragic implications: being rejected/cast out is viewed as an eternal sentence. Faults and flaws are not seen to be mitigated by circumstances, because things are judged as either all right or all wrong. Thus, as redemption is unlikely, punishment by exclusion is swift.

Even in traditions that stress love, forgiveness and grace, the underlying psychic atmosphere often feels like the childhood scenarios outlined above: Sincere people are doing their best to conform to external standards, while living in fear that the love they so desperately want will be denied them if they are not good enough.

Unrealistic Expectations

Our culture revolves around a series of unrealistic expectations for the shape of the body, and places a disproportionate value on sex appeal, and then manipulates our desires and exploits our deepest insecurities and fears. One look through any popular magazine or glimpse of a TV commercial provides ample evidence. Scroll through a yoga-dominated social-media feed and you'll find the same culturally-defined standards for beauty, happiness and success. These standards, moreover, promote not only the practice of yoga but the accessories to look the part. Skinny, white, supple, smiling women parade endlessly across the screens of our cell phones, tablets and computers reminding us again and again that who we are just doesn't quite have enough of that *certain something* to be valued and validated.

The game of "good enough" is rigged against us from the beginning, as long as we remain ignorant to the game's inherent futility. *We cannot win* against the systemic hypnosis of the culture's standards and perceptions of perfection. No matter how hard we try to meet the mark, we will inevitably fall short of perfection, resulting in an imagined loss of love, or the reinforcement of the fear of losing it. This dynamic functions like an addiction.

When we create such a relationship to perfection and love, our day-to-day lives are painful. Spilling over into our spiritual work, however, yields disastrous consequences. As the notion of perfection comes with us into the practice of yoga, we strengthen the misery many of us came to yoga to heal.

Yoga teachers, schools and communities often recommend practices and perspectives that are helpful during certain stages of our growth. Perhaps, we commit to a regular schedule of classes, adopt a breathing practice, learn to recite a mantra and/or sit in meditation. Perhaps, we moderate our diet, regulate our sleep and study inspiring texts and scriptures. These are wonderful protocols that can bring sanity, clarity and stability into our lives and can alleviate the suffering coming from a lack of awareness or various self-indulgent patterns. For instance, one sure-fire way to avoid feeling hung over every morning is to stop drinking so much! Common sense can take us a long way. Of course, anyone who has dealt with obsessive, compulsive patterns also knows that "just saying no" is not always easy or straightforward.

Rules, standards and expectations for being a "good yogi" can be found in all domains—from frequency of practice, to poses, to diet, to inner serenity—and expand exponentially once we start teaching yoga. Sincere practitioners often feel that if they came to their mats *every* day, instead of only three or four times a week, they would be better yogis. Or, if they were vegetarian, alcohol-free, sugar-free, gluten-free, etc., they would have such a "clean" diet that they would be cleansed of their perceived flaws and faults.

Sometimes, perfectionistic tendencies grab hold of the postural practice and convince practitioners that—if they were stronger, more flexible, more open, more stable, more intelligent, more dedicated— they could accomplish those ever-elusive poses and thus be better yogis. I could go on endlessly with examples, but the important point is how easily perfectionism can dress up as yoga practice and continue to reinforce the very beliefs we are hoping to heal.

The Trap of Self-Improvement

Nothing is wrong with wanting to expand and improve ourselves. Many of us came to the path of yoga with life-threatening addictions and energy-depleting habits making us and those around us miserable. We came to yoga to have a better life. We came to yoga to improve upon our situation. We wanted to hurt ourselves and others less. These are admirable aims and worthy motivations. We can and should do what helps us and benefits others. Sane lifestyle choices that improve the quality of our daily life and relationships are part of the foundation on which we build a life of practice. The work of change is critically important . . . up to a point.

However, after that point, self-improvement becomes a trap of its own. Yoga protocols and practices have a way of strengthening conventionally-determined notions of perfection, rather than loosening them. While practices can help us recognize our essential wholeness, commonly we engage in them from a self-improvement context. Then, doing that same practice day-in and day-out, year after year, may only serve to remind us that "something wrong" exists within us, or that we are not complete yet, and thereby undeserving of love, belonging and vitality. Being a good yogi becomes the new standard for our worth, and we are taken on a ride down the same childhood road of "not good enough," not part of the family, and not able to meet the mark.

Built into even the most empowering self-improvement plans is the deep-seated belief that love is conditional, that it must be earned, and that it can be taken away. At some point on the path, even trying to be a good yogi will most likely become a source of suffering, disillusionment and disappointment.

This post-honeymoon stage of practice is profoundly important. The stark view of our situation—even when painful and humbling—invites us to move beyond our fantasies of yoga into a new stage of clarity, and into the reality of our life of practice. If yoga is about a direct relationship with reality, our fantasies about the practice will need to be exposed for what they are. And while this stage of growth is uncomfortable—full of disappointments and disillusionment—I believe it holds tremendous possibility. Luckily, there is no better way to learn unconditional self-love than to engage in a task at which we repeatedly fail. Shifting a lifetime focus away from *earning* conditioned love by pursing perfection, to a focus on unconditional love and self-acceptance, will not happen easily or quickly.

Love's Learning Process

The good news: Built into love's own learning process are the seeds of the heart's deepest virtues. The fact that the work will take some time teaches us patience. The fact that we can't figure it all out intellectually will help us learn what wisdom lives beyond the analytical mind. The fact that we will fail repeatedly will teach us humility. The fact that we will feel scared will teach us courage. In the midst of our difficulties, we will develop the qualities and skills we need to meet our challenges.

The disappointment that follows upon unmet expectations is the result of a pendulum-swing—back from the zeal of our new conversion to the disillusionment of finding ourselves as we are . . . unchanged in so many ways, yet more painfully aware of our predicament. The experience of this psychic-pendulum-swing invites us to our wholeness—to self-acceptance rather than perfectionism; to become the recipient of our own love, a love that doesn't rely on being perfect, changed or different from who we are. As long as we are bent on relentless self-improvement, unconditional love and full-hearted self-acceptance will elude us because our "more and better" efforts will strengthen deep patterns of self-hatred, self-criticism and self-loathing.

There is simply no way to open the doors to love and compassion without going through those things standing in love's way. At a psychological level—in the shadows of the disowned, disregarded aspects of self—small windows to our wholeness await opening. Spiritually speaking, we don't have to earn the love that is our true nature—that love already lives within us as the essential Self. We already *have* what we are trying to earn. However, plenty of work must be done to disempower the beliefs and behaviors blocking us from the recognition of the love that lives at the heart of who we are. And we cannot work on, or with, what we do not know about.

Fixing What Is Already Whole?

My therapist once asked me if I wanted to be perfect or if I wanted to be whole. At the time, I wanted to be "fixed" because I felt broken. I assumed "fixed" lay on the other side of "broken." I thought therapy and yoga would help me patch all the cracks, cover all my scars and turn me into someone without bad habits, insecurities, jealousies and personality quirks. And, truth be told, I figured being fixed was some form of perfection.

As I've learned from making this journey, "wholeness" is on other side of broken and flawed—not "fixed," not "perfection." On the path of wholeness, all of my brokenness—my cracks, scars, bad habits, insecurities, jealousies and personality quirks—are part of the tapestry I am weaving and give texture, depth and nuance to who I am.

A DEEPER YOGA

The salient difference between yoga as an inner journey incorporating a practice of wholeness and yoga as a self-improvement project, rests on our choice of a few fundamental assumptions: Are we unloved and unlovable, trying to earn love through practices that will make us more perfect and therefore more lovable? Are we bad, trying to get good enough to be loved? Or, are we essentially loved, using practice as a means to experience and express that love creatively and authentically? Is practice an effort to remove the obstacles to the field of love within us so we can reside there more consistently and make our choices from there more reliably?

Whether we have aligned with the self-improvement camp or the inner journey approach, the outer work of yoga may still look exactly the same: We may eat a wholesome diet, practice yoga asana, chant, practice pranayama, meditate, pray, etc. Or, maybe the external work will look quite different: We may let go of perfectionist expectations and learn to place fewer conditions on our own love, only to find that we don't seem as "together" as we used to—maybe we let our house get messier; possibly we gain weight, or maybe we don't practice asana every day. However, as the reference point of our yoga evolves from earning love and approval through self-improvement to recognizing, cultivating and expressing love as an inner orientation, a profound shift becomes available to us.

Once again, freedom and peace do not live in achieving or conforming to outer standards but in the recognition and experience of our inner wholeness. When we glimpse the fullness of who we are, we find that love is our true nature. New possibilities show up because we have created a new reference point for our relationship to ourselves, to our bodies and to our life of spiritual practice.

For me, understanding that being perfect was an impossible goal was both a relief and a conundrum. At first, the news was good: Being perfect is not required for love. *Hallelujah*!

However, on the heels of that bold assertion came the startling (horrifying?) recognition that I had spent my entire life working toward a myth. My type-A, driven, achievement-oriented personality was all constellated around a false premise. Even my life of yoga practice rested on my achievement-based neurosis and a false identity aimed at proving my competence to myself and others at every turn. Not one area of my life was untouched by this insidious belief. I had invested countless time and energy in the pursuit of an essentially false ideal, and even though the pattern caused me misery, the pursuit of the myth gave shape to my life. Letting go of perfectionism sounded great, but surprisingly difficult to do. After all, I was less practiced in, familiar and accustomed to, living without the ever-present psychic urge to "improve myself" and to "get my shit together" and to "show everyone how awesome I am." Furthermore, "muscling" this improvement process wouldn't fix the problem, because this struggling towards perfection was the problem in the first place. Instantaneous with this realization, moreover, being less perfectionistic could become my new self-improvement strategy—something to do well, to achieve and to overcome.

Where Freedom Really Lives

One of my yoga teachers tells a story of being with her guru in a meditation session. A hard-working, achievement-oriented type herself, she was sincerely doing her best to follow the meditation protocols as outlined by her teacher. One day, well into the meditation period, her guru called her by name and said, "You can't get after it from the mind, you know."

Of course, she tells the story fondly and with humor today, while admitting that, in the moment, she was mortified to be called out in such a direct way. The story illustrates the conundrum of healing perfectionism. Perfectionists tend to want to do things well. *Perfectly*, if you will. And, having identified a problem—such as being perfectionistic—a perfectionist will want to quickly fix the problem so as to be, well, *perfect*. But, perfectionism can't be fixed; it must be *lived into,* and consciously, so that the myth can be exposed, little by little, for what it is—a lie of the mind. And the only way to see a lie of the mind is to appeal to an authority that is higher or deeper than the limited, thinking self.

For me, unraveling the knots of these patterns requires ongoing soul-searching and the help of a good psychotherapist. As potent as meditation, mantra, pranayama and asana are, they may not be sufficient without the aid of a trained therapist who understands the interplay between spiritual growth and psychological development. This book is not meant as a substitute for psychotherapy, as an eating disorder treatment, or for psychological assistance of any kind. Instead, this book outlines a process to provide support for you in the unique journey you are on in relationship to your body, mind, emotions and spirit as a yoga practitioner.

I do not think psychotherapy can substitute for spiritual work and for the expanded states of consciousness yoga-inspired practices yield. However, researchers and educators in the fields of both spirituality and psychology are currently in dialogue, publishing and speaking about the importance of integrating both disciplines in meaningful ways. For modern day yoga practitioners who want to move beyond the traps of perfectionism and conditioned love, integrated psychological work can help spiritual growth tremendously.

In the next chapter we will consider the primacy of compassion in the healing of perfectionism.

Inspiration, knowledge and experience move into wisdom through integration and articulation. In troubling times, we are bombarded with information, misinformation and a cacophony of voices competing for our allegiance. We do not live in a time where the outside sources of information are always reliable or hold our best interests in mind. Learning to access, integrate and rely on our inner wisdom is not just an esoteric idea, but a survival strategy for times like these. Not just a vague principle or a good idea, the capacity to trust ourselves is immensely practical and immediately relevant.

—Christina Sell

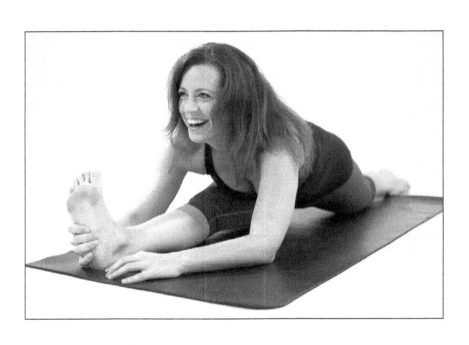

CHAPTER 4

CULTIVATING COMPASSION

———

Compassion for oneself is similar to compassion for other people. Compassion is the acknowledgement of another's suffering coupled with a sincere desire to alleviate that suffering in some way. When I consider the current condition of Western culture—systemic racial prejudice, gender-based oppression, and the ubiquitous marketing machine mercilessly preying upon our deepest fears and most tenderhearted desires—I often feel overwhelmed, as though the odds are stacked against us. However, my next impulse is to validate the difficulty and necessity of the work of self-love.

Self-compassion occurs when we can recognize, validate, and in some way "be with" our own suffering. The word "compassion" is made up of two parts: *com* meaning "with" and *passion* (from the Latin *passio*) "suffering." Compassion, therefore, means to "suffer with," and thus implies "*being with* suffering." So, for example, instead of finding fault with ourselves because we dislike our bodies or wish they were different, self-compassion allows us permission to "be with" that recognition, without judgment. Let's face it, given what we are up against in conventional society, it is likely that we would have some dissatisfaction with who we are, how we look, and/or how we feel. Is it any surprise that self-love feels distant, elusive and out of our reach so much of the time? Self-compassion is an antidote to perfectionism.

We need to actively cultivate self-compassion, which involves several choices and assertions. First, we make a choice to *see* our suffering—both the self-created forms and those that are part of our human condition.

Then we can assert that, while also personal to us, any suffering is part of a shared human experience. Some of the deepest psychological wounds people have (and therefore "suffer") are the mistaken ideas of "not enough" or "too much." And those notions sit right next to the sense of "not belonging" and being "different from"—or as the 12-Step communities say, being "terminally unique." Compassion for ourselves comes alive when we can see our own struggles (real or imagined) in the light of a larger story—part of a unique and shared journey of growth—as opposed to proof of our flawed nature.

For many people, this attitude of loving self-acknowledgement does not come naturally. Even the sincerest practitioners can be increasingly frustrated by trying to see themselves clearly, to say nothing of attempting to "be with" their suffering, simply allowing them highly uncomfortable feelings and agitated moods. In these moments of frustration and seeming futility, when even our best efforts do not appear to have yielded any fruit, we most need our own compassion.

> Instead of mercilessly judging and criticizing yourself for various inadequacies or shortcomings, self-compassion means you are kind and understanding when confronted with personal failings—after all, who ever said you were supposed to be perfect?
>
> —Kristin Neff

Beyond Positive Thinking

Cultivating compassion in the face of success and failure is one of the best antidotes to the toxic cycle brought on by any achievement-based perfectionistic expectations—those lures that entice us even in spiritual practice, ready to co-opt our wholeness and turn our efforts toward familiar conditioned patterns.

While learning new skills, mastering unfamiliar actions and achieving certain poses can and do build confidence and self-esteem, the price of accomplishment-based self-esteem is that we often feel worse when we cannot do something or when we encounter one of our limits. When this variety of self-esteem comes with us into the yoga room or onto the meditation cushion, it can keep us locked in the cycle of perfectionism where our value and worth is tied to our behavior and accomplishments, not referenced in our inner wholeness and essential fullness. Getting "better and better" will never free us from the trap of using outer reference points to define our worth.

Cultivating self-compassion, regardless of achievement, involves meeting ourselves where we are and becoming a friend to ourselves in our moments of suffering. When we turn our own loving understanding inward, we soothe ourselves from within, unleashing a flow of healing, empowering and kind positive energy. This approach should not be confused with using positive affirmations, whereby, in the face of any given upset, we attempt to assure ourselves of the opposite. For instance, if we feel fat, we might assert, "You are beautiful," or if we feel left out, we might say, "You are loved." While that kind of self-talk reversal can help, we also run the risk of feeling inauthentic or less than genuine in applying such affirmations. On the other hand, when our practice is about awareness rather than achievement, attention over improvement, and compassion instead of perfection, our relationship with ourselves becomes more balanced, truthful and mature.

Don't Try to Change

In a recent conversation with a friend of mine, I noticed myself feeling tired as I listened to her testimony of radical change and growth on the spiritual path. Don't get me wrong, I was happy for her, and impressed that she attributed her new-found freedom to her practice. But as she spoke, I was aware that, in my own experience, I was less interested in the pursuit of change and self-improvement, and more interested in how I was actually *living* alongside those things within me that, like it or not, had not changed.

I am not talking here about "living alongside" life-threatening addictions and abusive patterns of behavior. We *do* need to work on some issues for the safety of ourselves and others, and at several points in my own journey I needed to change if I was going to live. That sounds dramatic, but I am quite serious. I had some life-threatening behaviors that needed to stop. Believe me, I know how important shifting some patterns can be.

But I have stopped thinking some kind of salvation awaits on the other side of all the things "wrong" with me—whether those things are merely perceived or actual as judged by me or by others. I am talking here about the ten-thousand neurotic tendencies that annoy, distract and rob joy in ways too numerous to name. I am talking here about the things I hold against myself and use to keep self-love continually out of reach, turning my own regard into something I have to earn—a self-regard with the unrealistic price tag of perfectionist standards I will never meet.

Instead, I believe salvation is to be found *within* those tendencies and behaviors I hold against myself. That salvation is self-compassion. Not the surface-level compassion containing the often-unconscious promise of "one day I will change." But the compassion possible when I can truly *be with* my own suffering—my impatience, jealousy, frustration, anxiety, anger, shame and sadness—with no reassurance that "one day I will overcome."

Ironically, the salvation of my own regard and tenderness, of my own self-compassion, often creates a shift. This shift may not always be obvious in my outer behavior, but inwardly I know the shift as a re-direction of my attention toward love. That re-direction is one of the sweetest fruits of practice, and where my primary interest in yoga lies.

In practicing self-compassion, we don't seek to change our feelings of discomfort as much as to "make room" for them to exist *inside the field* of our own love, understanding and acceptance. We make room for the fact that postural practice, for all the help it can give us, can also be an achy, awkward foray into the stiff nooks and crannies of the body, mind and emotions. We needn't pretend otherwise. Meditation practice, for all its boons, is not always relaxing, blissful or easy. Sitting with the machinations of our own mind is often uncomfortable and difficult, which we don't have to deny.

Paying Attention

Sometimes we try to reassure ourselves something is true, even when it isn't "true" for us based in our current, honest, emotional experience. Instead, we can practice tuning into the "true"/felt sensations of our own body. Then, even feelings of upset or fear or anxiety become no more and no less than our embodied experience in the moment. In the grip of such fear and anxiety, we can learn to feel the sensations of our heart beating, our jaw clenching and our palms sweating. We can tune into our body as a way *to be* with our emotions without additional drama or minimization. This mindful approach to difficult emotions helps us walk the razor's edge of emotional work: Feelings do not get exaggerated or denied, but instead are directly observed, claimed, experienced and integrated.

Asana practitioners are well-trained in how to be aware of body sensations, and yet we often fail to apply this same awareness to our inner life of emotional and psychological development. Just like we learn how much stretching our muscles can take before injury by paying attention to the sensations of our body, we can learn to pay attention to the sensations accompanying our emotions to help us manage their intensity without overwhelm or denial.

One of the best ways to communicate to the people in our lives that we care about and value them is to pay attention to what they want and need. When we care about people, we make time to spend with them and plan activities together we both enjoy. Intimate friends know our soft spots and insecurities as much as they see our talents and strengths. A true friend stays the course through the ups and downs of life. In the same way, paying attention to ourselves is an act of friendship, intimacy and love that should not be disregarded.

For most of us, self-love will not come with bright lights and big bangs. Instead, a loving relationship with ourselves will evolve much like any other relationship in our lives—over time, with good days and bad, through joys and sorrows, and in both the mundane moments of ordinary life as well as in the peak experiences of revelation and grace.

Limits As Reminders

Whether we are considering asana or another contemplative practice like meditation or pranayama, we can expect to encounter our limits on many levels—physically, emotionally and intellectually. No matter how proficient we may be at asana, there will be poses we cannot do due to a lack of strength, flexibility, body proportions and our unique physicality. We will encounter emotional blocks to practice, and boundaries we need to set with our teachers, students, colleagues and friends. And, our understanding of philosophy, anatomy and the many nuances required to practice or teach may exceed our intellectual capacities along the way. The possibilities for self-criticism are endless, particular to each of us, and too numerous to name. Limits are to be expected in any in-depth study or any intimate relationship. A long-term practice is, in fact, a study involving many relationships—the most primary being the one we have with our self and our consciousness. And while I can state unequivocally that limits are to be expected, many of us will still feel ashamed, diminished in our self-esteem, when we reach a boundary. When we can recognize such shame, disappointment or self-criticism, we have the perfect moment for practicing self-compassion.

Instead of blaming a teacher for a pose that is too hard, or blaming yourself that you can't do a pose, understand a concept or feel differently than you do . . . what if instead you practiced the self-soothing ritual of being kind to yourself, acknowledging your common humanity and bringing mindful awareness to the moment? You might tell yourself something like: "You are doing the best you can do. That is a new and unfamiliar posture to you. A lot of other people struggle with these poses also. And really, this pose will be finished soon, and this upset will pass without needing to sweep you away like it is the most important thing in the world."

No matter how well our practice seems to be going, or how poorly, we can use any facet of reality *just as it is*, to move toward self-compassion. These sincere attempts to befriend ouselves will create an inner and habitual momentum. Instead of expecting life always to go our way, or to conform to our expectations or society's standards . . . and then beating ourselves up when we aren't perfect . . . we can develop self-compassion keeping us in a relationship to ongoing, personal and internalized love.

Suggestions for Practice

1. **Writing a Letter:** Identify a situation that triggers self-criticism or shame for you. As though you are corresponding with a friend in a kind and understanding way, write a letter to yourself expressing how you genuinely understand why you feel the way you do. Tell yourself other people feel the same way. List any specific examples you know of in which other people felt the same way.

2. **Self-Compassion Ritual:** Lie on your back. Place your hands over your heart. For 2-5 minutes offer yourself your own compassion. If you are having a hard time, make sure you acknowledge that fully. If you are feeling pretty good, let that be a doorway into greater positivity. Consciously encourage the outflow of love toward yourself as well as the flowing in of your own regard. Take time to be both the giver and receiver of your own self-compassion.

3. **Compassion Candle:** Create a small altar to signify your intention to become more compassionate with yourself. Place a candle on the altar, and light it every day. Breathe slowly into your heart while you watch the candle.

PART II

FOOD & OTHER HUNGERS

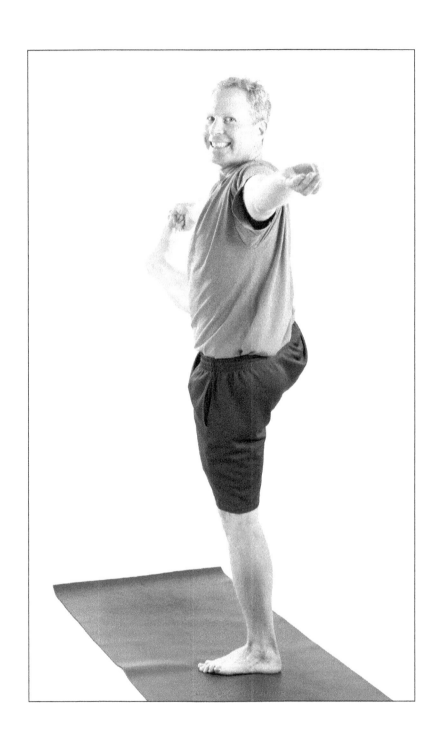

CHAPTER 5

ADDICTIONS & SPIRITUAL MALADIES

―――――――

When I was writing *Yoga from the Inside Out*, I interviewed my spiritual teacher Lee Lozowick about body image and spiritual life. I asked him what the relationship was between spiritual practice and a healthy body image. He stated boldly, "Body image has *NOTHING* to do with spiritual life."

My heart sank.

He continued, saying, "Spiritual life deals with seeing Reality *as it is*, not about improving our image of reality."

Lee's comment became a koan for me as I lived into the questions of how I might reconcile my body-image struggles with a life dedicated to spiritual practice and Reality *as it is*.

As a bulimic, my struggle with my body had life-threatening consequences. When I looked in the mirror, I did not like what I saw. The influence of the Sleeping World's standards of beauty had me in a constant state of self-hatred and anxiety as I tried to conform to something my body could never be or do. However, body image was only one facet of my struggle.

I was obsessed with food and diet, as are countless others in affluent culture. Yet, while I hoped some diet or food plan would work for me, I too was often rebellious, opinionated and resistant to making changes in my longstanding beliefs and habits around food. Vast numbers of the population exhibit the extremes of unhealthy thinness and eating disorders, while larger numbers are prone to obesity, which has hit epidemic proportions in the United States. Clearly, food is an arena where many of us struggle to find balance.

I am not interested in fat-shaming, or in preaching about the size and shape of other people's bodies. Rather my interest is in the addictive relationship to food that results in bingeing, compulsive eating and pacifying the emotions through food in ways leaving people feeling out of control, powerless and/or depressed. Food addiction is a serious issue, and I see excessive weight—to a degree that threatens health—as a symptom of an unbalanced relationship with food. Excessive weight typically indicates being out of contact with ourselves in deeper ways. Dieting, bingeing, purging and food restriction are all different facets of the same spiritual malady that I have been exploring throughout this book. The malady that my teacher Lee was pointing to—that of failure to truly see and embrace Reality, as it is.

My Story

I couldn't stop eating. Every day, I woke up and promised myself I would not binge or purge. Every day I binged. Every day I purged. Repeatedly. The binge and purge cycle went on for years in a torrent of demoralizing powerlessness that eventually took me close to suicide.

After years of bingeing and purging, I was out of touch with my physical body and its sensations of hunger and fullness. My body chemistry was disturbed so I was extremely sensitive to certain foods like chips, cookies and ice cream—so much so that even a small amount of these foods would trigger uncontrollable binges. For a while, I worked with a food plan as well as the 12-Step recovery program to help me find both a structured way to eat and a way to inventory and resolve the deeper issues that drove my obsession and compulsion.

I couldn't stop purging until I stopped bingeing. I couldn't stop bingeing until I addressed the emotional reasons for why I overate. I couldn't look at my emotions clearly until I stepped out of the arena where I was playing the game of outer image and outer validation. I had to get serious about the personal work of making peace with my body as it was, not with transforming my image of it. My life depended on it.

Deep patterns of unworthiness and fear lurked underneath the surface of my addictive process with food and my obsession with how I looked. Due to childhood sexual abuse, dysfunctional family dynamics and societal pressures, I focused on food rather than feelings; on appearances rather than my inner self. I used food much like an alcoholic uses alcohol—to numb my feelings, to relieve stress and to distract myself from the depth of my emotional pain.

I also used obsession with body image addictively. I criticized my body and felt shame about myself, rather than feeling happy, sad, scared or mad. Instead of feeling my feelings, I felt "fat," and then over-ate and purged to numb myself. Years of therapy helped me understand that "fat" is not an emotional feeling, and that underneath my worries about how I looked were deeper fears of not being lovable, safe, understood or valued for who I am.

One of the practical assumptions that guided my recovery from food addiction was that the desire to binge, purge, diet, worry or obsess about food (or my appearance) was a signal that something else was going on. For many years, I followed a moderate food plan that helped me identify the urge to binge as a signal that my emotions needed tending. Instead of snacking mindlessly, bingeing, purging, I learned dozens of strategies to self-soothe: ways to explore my inner life, such as praying for help, meditating, calling a friend, going to a meeting, writing in a journal, reading inspirational literature, taking a walk, practicing asana, and so on. I also learned that when I was obsessing about how I looked, or feeling "fat," those same self-soothing strategies could help me arrest the obsessive thought process and direct my attention to a deeper level of emotional truth and a saner process of thinking.

It took me almost a decade of ongoing effort to find a more natural and easeful relationship to hunger and fullness, and for my body, mind and emotions to harmonize enough to eat a variety of foods without bingeing or overeating. While learning to stop eating when my body was full rather than when my plate was empty and being able to sit with the discomfort of not seeing mounds of food on my plate at every meal are simple skills for some people, they were victories of epic proportions for me in my recovery. As basic as it sounds, the dictum to "eat when hungry and stop when full" took me a very long time to actualize.

Issues for All of Us

Once my issues with food had stabilized, I still had a compulsive exercise issue to address, as well as internalized patterns of body shame, body dissatisfaction and body dysmorphia that I have already described in earlier chapters.

Food and exercise addictions vary considerably from substance addictions like alcoholism or drug addictions. Alcoholics cannot drink in a moderate way, and their recovery process revolves around creating a 100-percent alcohol-free life. The recovery process is similar to narcotics addiction. As difficult as abstinence is, alcohol and drugs are not required for living life. On the other hand, food and exercise are fundamental building blocks for living a healthy life in a body. Recovering from food and exercise addiction is like asking a drug addict to use their drug of choice three times a day and keep it in its proper perspective. Clearly, recovery is no easy task.

As we proceed in considering a deeper yoga, understand that you as a yoga practitioner need not consider your issues with food, exercise and body image as addictions for these lessons to apply to you as well. As long as you are alive, you are in a body and that body needs food and exercise. There will never come a time when you will *not* have a relationship with your body, with food and with exercise, even if that relationship becomes more loving, evolved and sane. Even as we deepen our inner life and detach from the obsessive identifications with image, we practitioners still need to tend to the care and feeding of our bodies intelligently, compassionately and lovingly. These are the terms of embodiment and, as such, these are also the very terms of our humanity.

But, What Should I Eat?

No one system of eating will work for everyone. In fact, the reasons we diet are quite varied. Some of us are overweight, some are underweight. Some people struggle with anxiety, others with depression. Some of us have health concerns requiring specialized food plans. Some live alone and have a simple quiet life; others live in the midst of great stress and interact with lots of people. People in colder climates will need different foods in mid-winter than those who live in the tropics. Variables are endless.

While I will not offer a diet plan, or make recommendations about specific foods in this book, I will assert that food—and more specifically one's relationship to food—is a seriously important area to review. After I wrote *Yoga from the Inside Out*, I got numerous phone calls and letters from people who had struggled with eating disorders and body image issues in much the same ways as I had. By phone, email or in personal conversations, we would talk about the book, sharing our similar and different stories and experiences. After a period of sharing, quite often the reader would say something like, "Yes, I know that self-love is important, but what should I eat?"

The questions would always jar me a bit. I would think, "I don't *know* what you should eat!" I wrote my first book to explain to myself and others that the problem (food, body image, eating disorder, self-hatred, etc.) was a spiritual dilemma and that no food plan or number on the scale or dress size was ever going to fix an essentially spiritual problem. In my opinion, the answer—the only lasting peace—will come from realizing we are asking questions such as "How can I get thinner?" and "What should I eat?" when we should be asking questions like "What is my purpose?"; "How can I serve?"; and "Does my life glorify God and honor the essential goodness at the heart of everything?"

Having said the above, I do know from direct experience that when my relationship with food is tipped to an extreme, it is difficult for me to contemplate higher concerns like service and devotion. And, because the question of *what to eat* is so often accompanied by a person's deep sharing about their own struggles, I know food is an important topic to address.

I also know from experience that the content of my diet does matter. What I choose to eat and not to eat can have a dramatic effect on my physical health, my weight and my general vitality, including my mental and emotional outlook. In many ways, the body is a chemical machine. Different foods affect the chemistry of the machine and its balance. Each one of us will be served to learn about that balance directly.

In addition to the "what" of food, I pay very close attention to the "why" and the "how much" of food. In fact, as time passes, I pay more attention to my portion sizes than I do to the types of food I eat, as I remain committed to abstaining from bingeing and overeating, but I am not interested in excessive restrictions or creating a list of "good" and "bad" foods. I do not believe foods are intrinsically healthy or unhealthy, and I believe the language of "clean" eating can trigger eating disorders and exacerbate food-related obsession by tying diet to morality and notions of puritanical perfectionism.

I do believe food can contribute to our health and I believe some foods have deleterious effects on our health. But many foods deemed "unhealthy" can be incorporated into a healthy, sane lifestyle and contribute to a full-hearted enjoyment of all of life's flavors and textures.

In the next chapter we will look at other types of "food" the body-being needs, asking ourselves the central question underlying our addictions and obsessions, namely, "What am I really hungry for?"

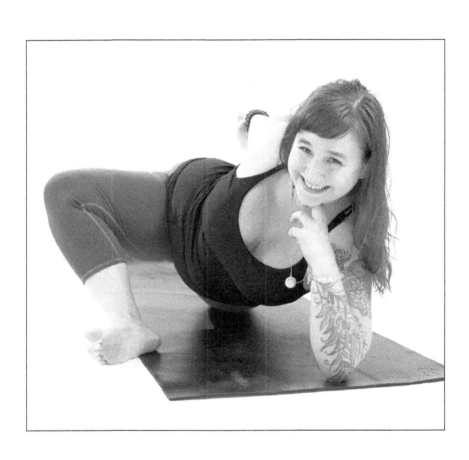

CHAPTER 6

WHAT ARE YOU HUNGRY FOR?

From a yoga perspective, our bodies are multifaceted, multi-layered and multidimensional. Simply put, we are physical, mental, emotional and spiritual beings. Different types of food nourish each aspect of us. Regardless of the content of your diet, you must crucially train yourself to understand and to respond appropriately to what I call "the four types of hunger:" physical hunger, intellectual hunger, emotional hunger and spiritual hunger.

The Four Hungers

Physical Hunger

Physical hunger is the hunger the body feels when it needs food or fuel. Just as a car needs gas to run, so too the body needs fuel in the form of food. Eating wholesome food free from chemicals and as close to its natural state as possible makes perfect sense.

Physical hunger also includes satisfying our taste buds so that we experience joy and pleasure in eating. Ideally, we find a balance in which we love what we eat as well as eat what we love. Both sides of the coin are important, and no success will come with a diet unless the food we eat is mostly satisfying and enjoyable.

However, our bodies are also hungry for other types of physical food, like movement and rest. We need water as well as food. We fail to thrive without appropriate touch. We need to gaze upon beauty, hear uplifting sounds and smell delightful and pleasing scents. We participate in our world through the senses and all they have to offer. The senses are part of our physical body. We are sexual beings. And while our work in yoga asana may move our attention inward, from the physical body to the energetic layers of reality, we will be doing that work in and through the vehicle of our body. The inner journey is not at the expense of the body, but instead uses the body to explore what lives within and beyond the outermost layer of who we are. If we deny, disregard or ignore some aspect of our bodies, some aspect of our wholeness will be left behind and the fullness of life will be truncated.

As I noted in the last chapter, I learned how to identify food-related aspects of physical hunger with the help of a structured food plan. After years of overeating and undereating, I had to learn about portion sizes, nutrition, and how different foods affected my energy levels, satiety and weight. Not to be confused with a rigid regime, a "structured food plan" was helpful for me to learn to identify the signals of true physical hunger.

Part of my long-term recovery has been to refrain from looking at foods as "good" or "bad," "healthy" or "unhealthy," or even labeling food as "clean." Rather than focusing on the specifics of each food we consume or abstain from, I see the "health" of our whole being as the result of many factors, notably including the effects of the foods we eat. Even a "wholesome diet" can feed obsessive, compulsive attitudes and behaviors, keeping us out of a direct relationship with our true physical hunger. Clearly, a steady diet of cookies and cake will not have good long-term effects. But expecting to live life with no sweets is probably unrealistic for most of us. Finding the balance that works for you as an individual will take time . . . and will most likely change throughout your life, depending on how your life circumstances unfold.

Additionally, there may be a time where you need or want to lose weight for a variety of reasons. While cultural standards of thinness are problematic, excess weight can cause strain on our joints and organ systems, and hamper participation in some physical activities. If, at some point, you choose to lose weight, it needn't be viewed as a result of fat-shaming (by yourself or others) or at odds with the principles I am outlining. I believe each of us, at different times in our lives, has an ideal physical expression. What I am pointing to here is not a fixed plan guaranteeing perfect weight and perfect health. Rather, I support you in becoming empowered to respond directly to what your body wants and needs.

Intellectual Hunger

Intellectual hunger is our desire for learning, for understanding and for tangible knowledge. Our intellect takes in information from our senses, then analyzes and applies the information to develop a body of knowledge that can guide us and shape our understanding of ourselves and the world. Any time we feel passionate about learning or about acquiring new information and skills, we are recognizing our intellectual hunger. Taking classes, attending lectures, reading books, writing, discussing ideas and concepts all satisfy this hunger for knowledge and understanding living inside each of us. When the intellect is not satiated through deep and meaningful pursuits, it will analyze, compare and typically judge situations and people harshly. The intellect is essential for navigating the complex world of culturally-determined ideals with clarity and discerning wisdom. Seeing beneath the surface-level of appearances is impossible without a well-developed intellect. The intellect compares, contrasts, makes distinctions, synthesizes, finds unifying threads of similarity and functions rationally.

True intellectual hunger differs from a compulsive drive to "have all the answers" or to "figure it all out." True intellectual hunger, when fed, can help give structure to our lived experience, can train our mind to work in our favor, and becomes an ally for growth and development in distinct contrast to just "being in our head." The desire to "get out of our head" often has to do with living too close to the mental machinations of fear, judgment and competitive comparison symptomatic of the culture at large. Intellectual understanding of our self-defeating patterns as well as our strengths can help us on the pathway to peace by keeping us clear-minded, discerning and focused on what matters most.

One of my teachers speaks in considerable detail about the "theory of the practice" and the "practice of the practice." The "theory of the practice" involves our intelligence so that we know how to best engage the work in front of us, and also how to assess the effects of our efforts. For instance, nutritional education can help guide our food choices and take the guesswork out of eating. Asana practice involves a tremendous amount of knowledge about the body, the postures, optimal sequencing and how to progressively approach the practice. In the same way, when we learn more about yogic principles, we can more readily shift our thinking and outlook toward other inspiring perspectives.

To move deeper than body image through yogic technology, we will need to educate ourselves about the distinction "what is *more than image*." And, "*what is more than the body only?*" If our education about the body has been primarily informed by the narrow understanding of modern society, we will need another and wider view. We need an ongoing education inspiring us to explore beyond the limited and painful relationship with body and image toward a more inclusive, empowering understanding of what is higher and deeper than cultural conditioning.

Yogic philosophy holds some common themes about body and mind that can be useful to study and work with. While some yoga traditions claim the body is an illusion, others see the body as a vehicle of the Divine, while another significant faction insists the body is an expression of Absolute Consciousness, albeit in contracted form. The shared principle in each system is that we are not our bodies and minds *only*—there is something else, something more. This something else or something more is knowable, and we need to learn the means and methods to come into relationship with it for ourselves. And while we cannot *think* ourselves into a new way of being, our intellect is necessary to understand the process of spiritual practice and to keep our bearings on the Path toward a greater freedom and a deeper orientation.

Emotional Hunger

Emotional Hunger is our hunger for authenticity, for personal expression, and for the instinctual knowing (non-rational but not irrational) beneath rational thought and analytical explanations. Our emotional nature is the source of our gut instincts and our heartfelt feelings, and contains a full spectrum of sentiments from anger, fear and sadness, to joy, exaltation and gratitude. When our inner emotional experience is observed clearly, it remains subject to our conscious choice about its expression. When out of our awareness, our emotions easily get blown out of balance, we often over-respond or under-respond. We get angry beyond what circumstances justify or we shut down and avoid engaging in relationships or life's various calls to action. Over time, without conscious awareness, patterns emerge that shape our emotional responses into habitual grooves, especially with regard to pain, betrayal and shame.

Emotional hunger, when unobserved and out of balance, can drive us to eat (or drink . . . or shop . . . or sex . . . or surf the Net . . . or text . . . or whatever) or cause us to withhold, withdraw from relationships or refrain from eating rather than feel our feelings. Sometimes we take a second helping of food (or a second/third drink, etc.) simply because it feels or tastes good, but many times we eat or engage in other forms of consumption more than what we require because an emotional discomfort arises when we are no longer engaged in the act of eating, for example. Where physical food is concerned, perhaps we feel awkward sitting at the table, finished with our meal, while other people continue to eat. (We can apply this same example of discomfort-relief to other types of activities as well.) That feeling of awkwardness goes away if we keep eating, so we continue eating instead of staying with our discomfort and moving through it, that is, until the emotional energy dissipates. Maybe we eat when we are at home alone instead of remaining present to our feelings of loneliness. Maybe we simply cannot endure the feeling of desire, the feeling of wanting some particular food or stimulation or contact, without acting on the urge. Or perhaps we refuse to eat enough or find health-based reasons to restrict our food consumption to feel control or to assert some kind of power over ourselves or our environment. The variations to this theme with regard to eating are endless and extend into all other areas of emotional need as well. But the point is, we can learn to recognize and respond to emotional signals to eat (or drink, or shop . . . or not eat, etc.) as distinct from physical signals. We can learn to understand emotional signals needn't be imperatives upon which we must act. Emotional hunger cannot be fed with physical food, with more friends on Facebook, or with more cosmetics or shoes. Emotional hunger must be fed by honestly acknowledging our emotions and by working with them and/or expressing them in healthy ways.

A fundamental premise of working with emotional hunger is there are no "good" and "bad" feelings. Anger is not less yogic than joy, nor is sadness less evolved than happiness. Feelings are *real* at the level of sensation and have essential information for us, if we want an authentic, intimate relationship with ourselves. Feelings are *not always real* at the level of circumstantial reality. For instance, I may judge or even perceive myself as fat, ugly and unloved by others, thereby giving rise to inner attitudes and sensations I then label as my "feelings." And those attitudes and sensations are currently "true" in terms of my experience of myself. But those "feelings" may not be "true" or accurate in terms of some objective criterion, or even how I look or seem to others, or how other people actually care about me.

What Are You Hungry For?

The Way Out Is In

My spiritual teacher used to describe the spiritual path as a series of interconnected, locked rooms. Each of us is, metaphorically speaking, locked in a room of our current state of being—physical, intellectual and emotional. The key to the next room, the next stage of growth, is hidden somewhere in the room in which we currently find ourselves. For instance, if I want out of a room of anger and upset, the only way to the next room is to discover what the anger and upset are telling me. I can pretend I am out of the anger room in countless ways—overeating, acting out, binge-watching TV, etc; but, the truth is, I will keep finding myself back in the anger room through repeating cycles of inner and outer circumstance until I can locate the key. Learning to be emotionally honest about the room I am actually in will help me discover the key to the next room. For instance, if I listen closely enough, sometimes I can hear the voice of longstanding resentment over past hurts. Other times, I find that my boundaries have actually been violated, or that I am replaying a scenario of being betrayed. Or perhaps, the anger sits on top of wellsprings of grief and sadness.

Learning to validate our full range of feelings (such as anger, sadness, fear and happiness) and to distinguish these essential ones from the mind-created judgments masquerading as feelings (unloved, betrayed, fat, ugly) is an essential part of moving our yoga from the surface toward the depths of who we are. Whenever we can both accept our feelings and see our self-judgments for what they are, using their signals to learn more about ourselves, we engage intimacy and friendship with ourselves. The more we do this, the less we are dependent on the outer world to accept, validate and bolster us.

I do not expect myself or anyone else to be 100-percent self-validating and not to care about other people's opinions. For me, such an ideal seems entirely self-referenced, and goes against much of our human experience, which relies on others in so many ways. However,

I do believe we can learn to do over fifty percent of the job for ourselves, thus freeing us from chronic emotional dependency on others.

Our maturity as yoga practitioners depends on some measure of self-sufficiency. No matter how kind and loving our teachers, friends and helpers on the path may be, they are simply not able to fill a need that we do not actively work to fill for ourselves. With respect to body image, if we can't be kind to ourselves, we won't be able to fully experience the kindness of others and will eventually conclude our teachers and community have "hurt," "betrayed" and/or "dismissed" us. No one can do this work alone nor can anyone do the work for us. Our emotional health and growth require learning to genuinely distinguish our feelings from our conclusions about our situations, and learning to feed emotional hunger in life-affirming ways.

Spiritual Hunger

Spiritual hunger, the longing we have for a life of dignity, joy and true purpose, leads us to serve something greater than ourselves, to realize our true nature and to allow our small concerns to be subsumed by a larger vision. Spiritual hunger aims toward fulfilling our highest ideals.

Spiritual hunger drives us to prayer, to acts of devotion and to moving beyond our comfort zone in order to satisfy a profound craving. Like emotional hunger, spiritual hunger cannot be satisfied with a second helping (or even a gallon) of premium ice cream, or a closet full of designer clothes . . . and so on. Even the best chef in the world cannot make a meal rich enough to fill us up in this way, nor could a vast inheritance of wealth. We must feed spiritual hunger with what will be most ultimately satisfying.

While some of us may relate easily to religious aims, including an involvement in formal spiritual schools, many others are fundamentally at odds with these structures. For spiritual hunger to be satisfied, we must engage our longing to know the greater wisdom of life in ways that feel true and authentic to us, while maintaining an open curiosity about what is yet unknown. Sometimes, our reactivity or recoil to a particular person, structure or system needs to be heeded—it may well be a sign that we are not in the right place at the right time. In other situations, the discomfort we feel may be due to unfamiliarity, inexperience or a perceived threat to our inner status quo. Remaining mindful, honest and interested in our inner experience is essential on the spiritual path.

A Deeper Yoga is not concerned with recommending any prescriptive religious or spiritual path. Instead, the book is an invitation to pay attention to the fullness of who you are, as you are, as an embodied affirmation of self-trust. Each of us needs to find the most authentic, effective and resonant streams of inquiry, experience and expression of our spirituality by referencing what is most universal within us. A spirituality that asks us to disregard our basic temperament will eventually create an unsustainable inner conflict. And yet, engaging a life of practice will change many aspects of who we know ourselves to be along the way. Knowing ourselves is only possible when we tell ourselves the truth, insofar as we can assess it, and learn to listen to what is highest and deepest within us. The best place to start—in fact, the only place to start—is from where we are right now.

Practicing Wholeness

In the same way that the body functions well with fresh, wholesome food lovingly prepared and presented, our intellectual, emotional and spiritual bodies function best when they are fed what they most hunger for. When we are not nourishing ourselves directly, we will feel empty and be easily susceptible to all of the damaging and degrading messages that the Sleeping World is selling us.

Additionally, as we recognize the different hungers within us and learn to respond to them appropriately, we will often highlight the interdependence of all aspects of our wholeness. That is, how our physical hunger and our spiritual hunger relate to each other or serve as checks and balances for one another. For instance, we will not want an exercise regime for the body that asks us to go against good, common sense, or one that is emotionally demeaning. We will not want to have a spiritual practice that asks us to ignore our body, avoid our emotions or abandon reason. By incorporating the whole of who we are in our endeavors, we can live fully—in an integrated, complete way—and avoid many pitfalls.

Suggestions for Practice

I. Checking in with the Four Hungers

1. Sit comfortably on the floor or in a chair. Close your eyes and focus on your breath. Imagine your breath moving throughout the length, the width and the depth of your body. Tune into your physical body. Ask your physical self, "What are you hungry for?" Wait a few moments to discover if a thought, feeling or inner message comes to you. If you get an answer, write it down.

2. Bring your attention to your thoughts and to your mind. Sit quietly and simply let thoughts arise without trying to enhance or suppress them. Observe the content of what you are thinking. Note how you may be analyzing something, planning, replaying memories, fantasizing. Ask your intellectual self, "What are you hungry for?" If you get an answer, write it down.

3. Follow the thread of your breath from your head to your heart and to your belly. Tune into your heartfelt longings and desires, as well as your sensations and gut instincts. Notice the mood of what is there: fear? sadness? joy? anger? Allow these feelings, longings, desires, sensations

to just be there, to be what they are, without any judgment or interference. Ask your emotional self, "What are you hungry for?" If you get an answer, write it down.

4. Bring your attention to the region of your heart and tell yourself that you wish to sink down into your "Spiritual Heart," imagining it like a chamber of white light within you. Here, where your highest vision lives, tune into your spiritual self. You may not have a clear reference point for what this means but relax anyway allowing whatever sensations and internal images may present themselves to arise. Ask your spiritual self, "What are you hungry for?" If you get an answer, write it down.

II. Imagine yourself free from your current doubts, fears, judgments and self-criticism.

1. How does it feel to be in your body without those judgments?

2. How might your life shift if you were not consumed with body obsession, food addiction or imposed constructs of improvement?

PART III

HEALING TOOLS

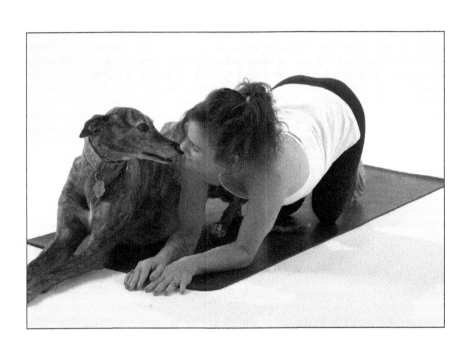

CHAPTER 7

TOUCHSTONES OF TRANSFORMATION

What I call "touchstones of transformation" are markers within life serving as important reference points for self-understanding. These touchstones—which might be particular energies, people, places, activities or events—help us break through conditioned patterns of limitation. They range from an expanded understanding of beauty, to the engaging of simple acts of devotion and love, to many other ways of bringing a refined quality of yogic insight into our daily lives.

Beauty

We begin this chapter with a consideration of a fundamental touchstone—beauty. Even with more diverse expressions of "a beautiful body" filtering into the media today, for instance, we are still going to be bombarded with images and messages that will fill us with self-doubt and shame. A deeper yoga practice, when it directs our attention inward and taps us into our elemental truths, provides us with an ongoing source of strength larger and more powerful than hollow, cultural imperatives.

> You don't have to be pretty. You don't owe prettiness to anyone. Not to your boyfriend/spouse/partner, not to your co-workers, especially not to random men on the street. You don't owe it to your mother, you don't owe it to your children,

you don't owe it to civilization in general. Prettiness is not a rent you pay for occupying a space marked "female."

—Diana Vreeland

Years ago, I rummaged through a box of old photographs I found in the basement of my parents' home. As I looked through the stacks of pictures from my childhood, I was touched by how adorable I looked. I took the pictures upstairs and asked my mother, "How did I grow up not knowing how cute I was?" She said she didn't know.

A few days later, however, Mom walked into my room and told me she had been thinking about my question. "I was a budding feminist at the time you were born," she explained. "When I was a girl, we were raised to be beautiful and to get a good husband. I wanted you to know that you were smart, capable, funny, athletic, independent and confident, not just beautiful. I must have forgotten to tell you that you were cute and pretty in my efforts to help you know that you were more than that."

The first time I remember feeling beautiful was during this same period of my life. I was on a wilderness expedition in Joshua Tree National Monument, miles from civilization, days since my last shower with no mirror in sight and setting up camp for the night. Making dinner with one of my favorite counselors, Dean, we were laughing hysterically about something that had happened during the day. Without warning the feeling struck me: I felt beautiful. In that moment, I was clear of the culture's ideals and free of the shame that had ruled my life. I felt 100-percent "beautiful," just as I was.

That same "free and clear" feeling happened when I first came to yoga in 1991. I didn't feel beautiful *during class*, mind you. Much the opposite. My first teacher was long, lanky-limbed and wore white unitards. She had a sinewy, classic "yoga body" . . . so common of the hippie practitioners of the time. She and others had been tying themselves in knots since around the time I was born, and hadn't had a hamburger since before the Vietnam War. I was twenty-two years old and probably twenty-five pounds heavier than I am today. I spent most of my first class feeling short, stocky and . . . let's just say it, *fat*.

Despite all that comparison and self-judgment, I remember getting up from *savasana*, walking down the hill to breakfast after class and feeling beautiful. Radiant, even. I can still recall the calm, tingly feeling I had in my body and the certainty that I had found something important for myself. I had found a beauty deeper than the size of my thighs, and a connection to who I was deeper than my appearance and deeper than what others thought about me. I had experienced my *prana,* my energy, and glimpsed an expanded reference point for self-understanding.

These expanded reference points are touchstones available on the journey of growing our yoga deeper than the body only, and deeper than body image. In the same way that my mother had wanted me to know that I was more than my appearance, yoga practice can help us stay connected with the part of ourselves that is more than appearance and more than the body only. We can come to know and value ourselves as compassionate, funny, strong, vital, sensitive and courageous, not just beautiful. Personally, I want my asana to be about how I feel in my body and not about how my body looks and who validates my appearance as beautiful or not. As a teacher, I want to be valued for my depth, my insight, my knowledge, my clarity, my hard-won wisdom and not for how good I look in a pair of tights.

Clearly, none of this work is easy because so much of life seems perfectly designed to bring us into the realm of our "something-less-than" or our "something-not-enough-as" instead of the realm of our "something-more-than." As I have referenced throughout this book, even in a pursuit as positive as yoga practice, we can fall prey to the pull of our negative, conditioned patterns. Identifying the internal and external forces acting on us will help us to recognize *when* we have been made a hostage of our self-defeating patterns of thought, feeling or behavior.

Still, the answer to moving beyond conventional notions of beauty and beyond our body-centered identification is not solely in the analysis of the issues at hand. Rather, such movement requires that we directly experience (i.e., be truly present to) those expanded states of consciousness. When such a state arises, we can affirm this beauty is our birthright, an interior state of being having nothing to do with what poses we can or cannot do, how we look, how we feel about how we look, or how we think other people feel about how we look.

Early in my recovery from bulimia, I surrounded myself with alternative and diverse images of beauty—dozens of visual impressions. Even in my house today, I have beautiful art—paintings, drawings and photographs—depicting women of all sizes and shapes, all reminding me that the female form expresses itself uniquely across cultures and times. As years have gone by, I have also expanded these images of beauty to include images and icons from a variety of religious traditions. By consciously acknowledging sacred representations of beauty, I believe I can imprint my consciousness with the sacred, giving me access to a field-energy beyond my conditioning. Surrounding myself with beautiful and sacred images can, in small and large ways, remind me of what is truly beautiful within me.

At the same time, let's be honest. I see no need for everything about our physical being to be related to as beautiful. In the spirit of the compassionate self-honesty I have been advocating throughout this book, if you do not think your body is beautiful, don't pretend. For instance, I have stretch marks on my thighs and I do not find them beautiful. I don't find them disgusting, either . . . nor do I feel shame about them. It would be a lie, however, for me to say I find them beautiful. In a sense, I'm simply neutral about them now. I don't need everything "all beautiful" in order to love myself, to practice compassion for myself and to feel worthy inside myself.

Whether it is weight gain or loss, aging skin, greying hair, cellulite, stretch marks, curly hair, straight hair, thin thighs, big thighs, curves or no curves, or even a nose you wish was different, I encourage you to engage the processes we've noted throughout this book. To summarize:

1. Cultivate a more inclusive and expansive perspective about yourself, affirming diverse forms of beauty.
2. Learn to recognize and validate this diversity as it takes shape as you.
3. Remember that who you *most truly are* is not tied to your appearance or to your feelings about your appearance.
4. Accept that disentangling the identification with looks will not come by swapping a negative image with a positive image, or by telling yourself something is beautiful if you don't find it so.

To know your worth beyond the surface-level of beauty is the invitation to a deeper yoga.

Suggestions for Practice

1. **Write:** Write for 10 minutes using the prompt, "I feel beautiful when …"
2. **Create a Beauty Collage:** Compile quotes, images, photographs and even small objects. Arrange them creatively on a piece of poster board, or wood, or some recycled "something." Hang your collage in a prominent place in your home.
3. **Make a Beauty Altar:** Create a small altar somewhere in your home that has a few select images that remind you of your inner beauty. Once a day, light a candle and place it on the altar as a reminder of your desire to know your own beauty more fully.

4. **Compliment Someone for Their Beauty:** Once a day, give someone a compliment about something you see or feel in them that is beautiful. Make the compliment about a quality of their being or about a virtue like humor, compassion or integrity, instead of how they look.

Nature

> We are born into a magical world of sensory delight, our beings naturally tuned to our surroundings. We are part of nature, our senses connecting us to the whole like an umbilical cord, allowing us to commune with and be nurtured by the source from which we have sprung.
>
> —Lang Elliot

A connection to the natural world is a touchstone to a broader view always available to us. The sky, the sun, the wind, the rain . . . these can become our compass needles pointing to our "true North," no matter what else is happening or where we happen to live.

Spending time in nature is also a wonderful way to cultivate appreciation for beauty. Many of us live in metropolitan areas, indoors for most of the day, while spending hours viewing our world through a computer screen, smart phone or TV. Fast-moving impressions designed to program us according to the Sleeping World's imperatives of fear-based acquisition, competition and self-doubt bombard our senses. Nature, however, moves at a different speed and remains a living expression of harmony, collaboration and interdependence, giving testimony to the eternal cycle of life itself. Oak trees are no less beautiful than aspens; daisies no less valid than petunias. Tuning into the natural world provides valuable lessons in humility, grandeur and significance (or insignificance). As we gaze out at mountains, canyons, oceans and rivers, we can know both our connection to nature as well as our relative powerlessness in the face of it. We cannot control the tides, the currents . . . or even the blooming of a flower in the fields.

As much inner power and wholeness as yoga helps us feel and cultivate, as much choice as our consciousness-building practices provide us, we are still *part* of an interconnected web of energy and matter over which we have little control. Nature is a wonderful reminder of the beauty, powerlessness, grandeur and humility of our *part*, even as She continually invites us back to our own true nature, which is fundamentally beautiful.

Connecting with nature in a profound way is a practice that takes time. At first, we may feel uncomfortable or bored as our mind adjusts to a different speed and an unfamiliar type of stimulation. But even small doses of regular immersion in nature can yield great benefits. When we recalibrate our senses and align ourselves with nature's rhythm, we start to see, hear, smell and sense more natural experiences of beauty. We actually create a new reference point for what beauty is, where it is sourced and how to relate to it.

From a spiritual perspective, immersion in nature is a touchstone for an expanded interior relationship with what enlivens us and the world around us. At the heart of spirituality is the breath and the act of breathing—the word "spirit" comes from the Latin root, *spirare*, which means "to breathe" or breath. And, we all know that the simple act of opening the window or moving outside often encourages us to take a breath, and momentarily alters our perspective. The breath enlivens our bodies and animates our souls. Anytime we feel "brought to life" or describe something as "breathtaking" we are close to something essential and important. In those breathtaking moments, we are at the threshold of spiritual essence, at the source of true beauty. The more time we spend in nature, attuned to this breath of spirit, the less the powers of conventional society can seduce, control or coerce us. We will know what it means to be beautiful from *inside* Beauty itself.

Suggestions for Practice

1. **Nature Walk.** Take a walk in nature, with no headphones or cellphone to distract you. Walk and observe smells, colors and sounds . . . all existing together in a complex and respectful relationship.

2. **Find a beautiful place in nature to sit and breathe.** Don't do anything specific; open your eyes, your ears, all your senses to the beauty around you with the intention that it nourish you.

3. **Find a book, series of poems or an article by a naturalist author,** such as Anne Zwinger, Edward Abbey or Walt Whitman, and read it for inspiration. For me, the poetry of Mary Oliver is particularly inspiring.

The Guru

A person can be a significant touchstone—heavy and life changing even! The word *guru* in Sanskrit points to such a person, but also more. The word actually means "weight" or "weighty," as well as "teacher."

Guru is composed of two syllables: *gu-*, meaning darkness and *-ru*, meaning light. The *guru* can be understood as anything that has the weight or gravity to bring light to darkness, or clarity to confusion or knowledge to ignorance. Think about how often we say, "Wow, that really shed some light on the topic," or how we describe someone as "lit up" when they are inspired and fully engaged. If we know how to look, we can see the *guru principle* active in common, daily language.

Essentially, the guru is a function, not a person or a personality. The guru serves the function of awakening, of helping the student wake up to the truth of who they are, through a process of syncing up called "entrainment." If you put a large clock in the center of a group of smaller clocks, eventually the small clocks will sync up with the big clock. The root of the word "entrainment" is -*train*, meaning *to pull* or *to drag*, and in this case, the big clock pulls or drags the smaller clocks into the big clock's rhythm. Much in the same way, the weight of the guru's expanded consciousness pulls the devotee into a similarly expanded perspective. Ideally, such temporary alignment eventually leads the devotee to the realization of the same state in which the guru lives. This process does not mean the student is coerced, tricked or manipulated in a guru-disciple relationship, although there are plenty of stories of how badly things can go. We can also see the principle of entrainment in our day-to-day relationships when we feel light and happy around certain people and we feel anxious or depressed around others.

In my relationship with my spiritual teacher, I experienced the entrainment like an energetic loan—a feeling of love arose from within me with greater ease when I was around him. For years, I thought the feeling was due to physical proximity because, when I was around my teacher, my own state of consciousness would shift quickly and dramatically. I always compared the quality of this state-shift to that of ocean air, which is characterized by an abundance of negative ions. While negative ions exist in the air everywhere, more are found close to the ocean. Consequently, the air feels different. And, as a result of being in proximity to the ocean, you feel differently too. Being around my guru was like being immersed in the ionized ocean air of expanded consciousness.

And yet, over the last decade of personal exploration, I have dealt directly (and indirectly) with some of the shadow issues involved in having my spiritual life centered on a guru figure. Essentially, communion with an outer "form"—such as a guru—may be a reference point for an inner experience, yet, making the psychic leap from the outer to the inner, from externalizing love to internalizing it, is often difficult, fraught with perils and problems. Add in the challenge of involvement with a spiritual community surrounding the guru, and the opportunities for dysfunctional transference, projection and co-dependency grow exponentially.

That being said, I think the guru function is embedded into life, which is always communicating with us, always inviting us to expand our reference points, and always challenging us to grow into the truth of who we already are.

Practicing a yoga *deeper than the body* is essentially training ourselves to learn the language that life uses to wake us up to these enlarged reference points. When we don't speak the language of awakening, challenges are "problems" and setbacks are "failures," and the circumstances of life determine who we know ourselves to be. "Happiness" gets tied to the happenings of life, so to speak. But when we begin to speak the language of awakening, we begin to see that below the surface of these same challenges, the "problems" and "failures" are actually pathways for growth. Whether the outer circumstances of life are joyful or painful, pleasant or distasteful, we can learn to enter them more fully, more honestly and with a greater sense of acceptance and compassion. And in so doing, we can find that *we* are fuller, more honest and more acutely compassionate than we previously knew ourselves to be.

Whether we're referencing the personal guru or the impersonal principle of life's unfolding, our touchstones have a cumulative effect. For instance, one asana session is not life changing, but a lifetime of sustained practice builds a treasure-trove of inner awareness that is profoundly transformational. One meditation session is more likely to be more frustrating than it is beneficial, but a lifetime of tapping into one's inner resources of wholeness becomes a real, palpable and benevolent sustaining force. Growing deeper through yoga is not a quick fix, but is instead life's work, which uses the nitty-gritty of our unique life circumstances throughout the entirety of our life to get the work done.

> ## *Suggestions for Writing Practice*
>
> 1. In what circumstances do you feel an expanded point of reference for who you are? How do you integrate these experiences into your life consciously?
>
> 2. What or who, in your life, carries the weight of spiritual authority? What people, situations, or teachings help bring light to your darkness? Write about this.

Wishing the Best for Others

ॐ सर्वे भवन्तु सुखिनः
सर्वे सन्तु निरामयाः ।
सर्वे भद्राणि पश्यन्तु
मा कश्चिद्दुःखभाग्भवेत् ।
ॐ शान्तिः शान्तिः शान्तिः ॥

Sarve bhavantu sukhinah;
Sarve santu niramayah;
Sarve bhadraani pasyantu;
Maa kaschit duhkhabhaag bhavet,
Om Shanti Shanti Shanti

May all be happy;
May all be without disease;
May all enjoy prosperity;
May none suffer any misery.
Om Peace Peace Peace.

This prayer is a touchstone for me as it expresses my strongest altruistic intentions. In Sanskrit, *sukha* (*sukhinah* in the prayer above)

means "happiness" and comes from a root that means "to move toward."
Dukha (*duhkhabhaag* above) meaning "suffering," comes from the verbal
root "to move away from." From a conventional viewpoint, we often
think of happiness as "good things happening" and suffering as "bad
things happening." From a yogic perspective, however, happiness is the
movement toward what is essential, eternal and intrinsic. By the same
logic, suffering occurs when we are moving away from what is most
real within us. When we are in the throes of suffering with negative
body image, for instance, we are obviously moving away from what is
most essential and being drawn into the snares of conditioned images
and perceptions. Connecting to the inward-moving current will help
us alleviate our suffering by helping us move closer to our true self,
which is deeper than outside imperatives and culturally-conditioned
injunctions.

But, the prayer is not simplistic or naïve, merely wishing that "great
things happen for everyone." Rather, it is an invocation that all beings
move toward the innate truth of Being.

On the road to the recognition and integration of our essential
nature, however, we will encounter dukha. Each of us will experience
pain as unresolved psychic knots are exposed, even as we are nudged
along toward genuine honesty and humility. If we prayed that all
those necessary challenges "move away" from someone, he or she
might be denied the requisite insight to grow, and we might lapse into
codependent patterns of rescuing . . . or failing to respect another's
process. At the same time, witnessing the pain of growth, loss, and the
suffering that life brings is hard. Most people, with any measure of
sensitivity, feel heartbroken and outraged by simply watching the news
or reading a newspaper.

This prayer is not an easy one. Considering "What *is* true
happiness?" requires a deep dive within to uncover the authentic
wisdom to answer the question as fully and clearly as possible. The
old bromide, "If you have your health you have everything," is not in

that category of responses. Praying/wishing for healing for ourselves and others does not mean that the physical body survives, a sickness ends or a surgery fixes our problems. Eventually, the physical body will come to an end for each of us. I have a friend whose mother entered hospice recently. Her mother was mentally ill and their relationship was fraught with challenges for them both. My friend told me that as her mother's cancer progressed over the past year, they were able to have thoughtful, peacemaking conversations that were healing for them both. Her mother's physical body would soon pass, and yet a profound healing had occurred.

What if healing was not only physical but could be found in understanding, compassion, forgiveness, equanimity and the capacity to witness suffering over which we had no control? A prayer for healing, like a prayer for happiness, is no simple matter.

Additionally, this chant serves as a powerful touchstone by suggesting a remedy for the misery of the mind—any violent, vindictive, jealous, afraid or otherwise contracted interior state. Such contraction happens when you harbor a resentment about a past wound, when you gossip, belittle others in subtle and overt ways, discount the talents another person has, fail to see your own talents, and/or find it difficult or impossible to delight in someone else's good fortune. The list goes on . . . and each of us generally has a typical "Contraction MO" that it is worth getting to know, and with as much compassion as possible.

A prayer-touchstone provides an opportunity to shift our own consciousness through the outpouring of love, compassion and beneficent wishes for others and for ourselves. It is not so much that we *try to be different* when we find ourselves caught in a web of our own suffering, but that we give ourselves the chance to invoke a higher state of consciousness through entering the flow of love. The effort to align with the flow of love is worthwhile.

I have found that a great tool for managing resentments is to pray for the people I'm angry with. This work is not naïve—it does not preclude acknowledging when harm has been done, nor does it replace the need for accountability, appropriate boundary setting and all the good tools of healthy psychological functioning. The work of offering love and good tidings to others (which this touchstone does) is actually in our own best interest. We will be steered by the mood of what we are offering, rather than by the mood of anger and its venomous expressions. Healing ourselves through love, and offering compassion to difficult people, informs some deep work with loving-kindness.

Loving-Kindness Meditation

The following meditation begins with recalling a "being" we love deeply as the starting point for cultivating loving-kindness. The technique is simple:

1. Center yourself.

2. Bring your attention to your breath.

3. Imagine your breath moving all along the length of your body.

4. Imagine your breath moving all across the width of your body.

5. Imagine your breath moving throughout the depth of your body.

6. Invite yourself to your inner depths.

7. Using your active imagination, invite a being you love to come join you.

8. Enjoy the impressions of being with this being—person or animal, alive or passed—and let the feeling of goodness be as real and as vivid as possible.

9. Imagine all the good things you want for this being and repeat the phrases: "May you be happy, may you be peaceful, may you be healthy, may you live with ease."

10. Now add yourself to your circle of good will and repeat the phrases—"May you be happy, may I be happy, may we be happy together; may you be peaceful, may I be peaceful, may we be peaceful together; may you be healthy, may I be healthy, may we be healthy together; may you be live at ease, may I be live at ease, may we live with ease together."

11. Let go of the image of the other and be with yourself. Repeat the phrases: "May I be happy, may I be peaceful, may I be healthy, may I live with ease."

12. Place your hand on your heart.

13. Offer yourself your good will.

14. Practice letting your own good will in.

15. Slowly deepen your breath.

16. Open your eyes.

Over time, as you grow comfortable in wishing loving-kindness to yourself and your loved ones, you can challenge yourself by inviting a difficult person into your inner space and offering them the same heartfelt intentions of happiness, peace, health and ease.

Cultivating the Mood of Love

Love lives at the very heart of my spirituality. My primary practice is not asana, meditation, mantra, pranayama or writing, but the cultivation of mood, or *bhava*. From this perspective, spiritual practice is not so much about attaining anything overtly holy or other worldly, nor is spiritual practice aimed at perfecting psychology, or getting the physical body whipped into shape. Practice is about removing my own conditions on love so I can see myself and the world without filters, demands and projections. The cultivation of mood, as a practice, is the conscious and ongoing *choice* to direct my attention toward love, love's source, and love's most optimal and authentic expression in my life. At the heart of spiritual life, for me, is not a perfect diet, an everyday outer ritual, or a laundry list of things to and not to do designed to reform my outlook, behavior and/or appearance, but is instead a movement toward love with love. This mood of love is the practice and the goal, the shelter and also the storm.

When I say "yoga," I am referring to those practices inspired by the yoga tradition in India as well as by my Western Baul spiritual teacher, Lee Lozowick, that give me a framework allowing me to discover and thus know who I most truly am. I do not claim my work is "real yoga" or "unruined" or "pure." I am a synthesizer, following in the footsteps of a crazy wisdom guru who used a variety of means to help me experience the grace of love. I am not on my particular path because I planned it this way in advance. Had I planned my path logically, I would have wanted a guru who was more politically correct, who gave less cryptic teachings, and who would not die of cancer before he was seventy. While I was at it, I would have planned to find an asana teacher to grow old with, not one with whom I would part ways when I was forty-two years old, after almost twelve years of study.

But I did not go about any of this work in a measured or calculated way. I jumped into the middle of the ocean of my own yoga experiment without carefully previewing my options, knowing the terms of study, and without realizing how deep and vast were the waters. I jumped in with a whole heart, desperate to save my life, needing to find a way to connect the longing I felt with the way I was living. I found a current of grace though my teacher and I have been swimming on that current to the shores of my own understanding ever since.

"Dog" Is "God" Spelled Backward

While writing the first draft of this book, drawing heavily from my previous book, *Yoga From the Inside Out*, I took a break to meditate. That's when I heard my dog, Locket, whining at my door. I let her in, hoping she would settle on the rug in front of my puja shrine so I could continue to meditate.

No such luck.

She whined. And whined. And whined.

When I opened my eyes and looked at her face—so full of expectant love and joy—I laughed. I had just been writing about spirituality, about the function of a guru, and about how love can be a touchstone for growth and change. My dog's arrival, and insistence on connection and play, was an immediate reminder of how ordinary the transforming force of love can be. Her request for my attention was undeniable . . . and for me, impossible to refuse.

If you knew me even a little bit, you would know how much I love my dog, Locket. I adopted her as a three-month-old puppy from a local rescue organization. Her playful exuberance and doting affection woke me up to something tender and delightful . . . something years of practice and inner work had not. We spend hours together hiking, biking, playing in the yard and simply being together. She often sleeps on a rug right next to me as I write or meditate.

On that particular morning, as we played, it dawned on me that a lot of my previous writing was like a pair of clothes no longer fitting me entirely well or suited me in style. I had outgrown many aspects of my previous perspective, and trying to re-use that same material was simply not going to work. I still agreed with the overall context of what I wrote almost ten years ago, but the tone and tenor were not as relevant for me now, nor applicable for this current writing project. Being steeped in a guru-yoga tradition for so long, I feel an immediate connection to love as expressed in the form of my teacher. I fall very easefully into that expression of devotion, as I acknowledge that my teacher has served me well. And this element of my previous perspective, which I referred to throughout the other books, remains true.

However, my personal process of integrating my experiences with my teacher and spiritual community with my own psychological development has required soul searching, truth telling and the reclamation of my own spiritual authority. While the love I experienced with my teacher remains a fundamental access point and expression of my spirituality and faith, the *terms and expressions* of that relationship have shifted significantly. My own interests now involve less focus on the "spiritual," or on my teacher, and more focus on the here and now of my life, as it shows up in every moment, with a view to enhancing my own authenticity and wisdom. In interrupting my period of meditation and turning the formal "practice" time into a game of fetch, my play with my dog captured the mood of these changes perfectly.

Many of these changes in my relationship to my teacher and to my own spirituality are natural outcomes of growth and development on the path of inner work. In retrospect, even though he suggested protocols and practices and had strong opinions about the optimal context for studentship, my teacher was always pointing me back to my own wisdom, clarity, and capacity to discern what was best for me. As time has passed, my experiences with him have integrated in such a way that the distinctions between the inner and outer teacher, the guru as person and the guru as a function, and even spiritual life versus ordinary life are more internalized, holistic, and personal than in my early days of studentship with him.

Practitioners of any yogic modality from asana to meditation can expect to find this kind of individuation process at work in their own life of study and practice. Many protocols and perspectives useful in the early stages of practice may shift organically over time as a result of new life circumstances, inner insight, and the various ways the practices and protocols advance and deepen our understanding of who we are and where we are aimed. For instance, one of my students is a recovering alcoholic. In her first few years of recovery, she went to an AA meeting every day and talked to her sponsor every morning and every evening. After twelve years of continuous sobriety, she doesn't practice the same way today as she did in the beginning of her journey. Now, she attends two meetings a week and talks with her sponsor much more occasionally.

In the same way, many asana practitioners and teachers spend long hours working on postures, learning anatomy and developing their teaching skills only to find that after many years, while they still love the practice, they no longer want to spend so many hours of each day devoted to it in the way they did initially. These inner and outer shifts are not always a sign of a lack of interest in practice or a devolution in one's growth, but may instead point to a more integrated, internally-oriented relationship to the tools and techniques of the path. For yoga to be a life-long relationship seeing us through the many seasons of our life, we must be able to allow the mechanisms of our relationship with yoga and our attitudes about ourselves and our practice to grow, expand, and change along the way.

Later on during this day when I had chosen to play with my dog, my husband told me something similar had happened to him in the morning. Up early to meditate and write in his journal, as soon as he sat down, the cat jumped on his lap and got settled on his notebook. When he looked outside, the sunrise was glorious. After a few futile attempts to move the cat off his journal so he could write, he decided to just be there with his cat and in the glory of the rising sun, with his heart and his eyes wide open. Life was unfolding in radiant splendor and with the loving presence of his cat in his lap he said it seemed unnecessary to close his eyes in order to experience something sacred. All the goodness he could hope for was right there in front of him.

These outer examples remind me that people, pets, places, things and activities can be beloved to us, and that "spirituality" or "practice" needn't be esoteric, cultish or outside the domain of our daily life. The *direct experience* of love in the outer world can soften hard edges around the heart, help relax the cynicism of the mind, and allow for an opening to an enriching, satisfying and nourishing embodied joy and connection. When love is fully expressed toward something external, that love can be a touchstone for transformation.

Let's extend this discussion of love-as-a-touchstone to cultivating a deeper yoga. One of the gifts of asana is, after a practice session, we often feel better than we did when we started. How many times have you gotten up from *savasana* feeling lighter, clearer, relaxed and more energized than when you began? Feeling better in our bodies gives us an expanded experience of our body deeper than image and appearance, because the feeling is referenced internally, in our direct experience of feeling good. Over time, "feeling better" can become an internal reference point for love. We walk through the doorway of simply feeling better straight to the heart of where better is sourced— inside ourselves, in the field of love. No matter how good or how bad outer circumstances are, no matter how affirming or negating the media are, no matter how brilliant or flawed our teachers are . . . our feeling-responses to any circumstances, media and teachers are inside of us. Therefore, we have choice in that domain.

This ability to choose how we will relate to life is not to be confused with some new-age cliché that "we create our own reality," which commonly gets mixed into the narrative of consciousness exploration. I find it deplorable that the idea of having choice in our feeling responses get twisted, and is used to rationalize harmful, disrespectful behavior: For instance, saying to others, "If you feel hurt by what I've done, then it is your story; your upset has nothing to do with me." Understanding that the source of our experience is internal does not give license to ignore our responsibility to others, nor should the principle be used as a means to avoid accountability for the motives behind, and/or consequences of, our actions. Assuming the source of positive and negative feelings lives within us does not mean other people do not affect us or that we do not affect them. In fact, the closer we come to our true nature and the more deeply we reference our lives in Love and compassion, the more likely we are to see how much we influence one another and the less likely we are to want to harm others.

Suggestions for Writing Practice

1. Which of the Touchstones noted in this chapter has the most power and attraction for you at this time in your life: Beauty, Nature, Guru, Prayer, the Mood of Love? Take 10 minutes and write about that one: For example, "Beauty for me is about ..."

2. In your imagination, "walk" through your home, and/or review a typical day or week, noting what Touchstones you have determined to use or have available to you. For example: your weekly tea date with a close friend; your use of flowers; work in your garden, etc. Take 10 minutes and write about how this Touchstone supports you.

3. Make a list of friends, family and people you admire, noting the Touchstones each of them seems to have a relationship to. For example: Aunt Dorothy who uses classical music to begin and end each day. Look over the list and note what this reflection inspires for you. Write about this experience: "As a result of this list writing I ..."

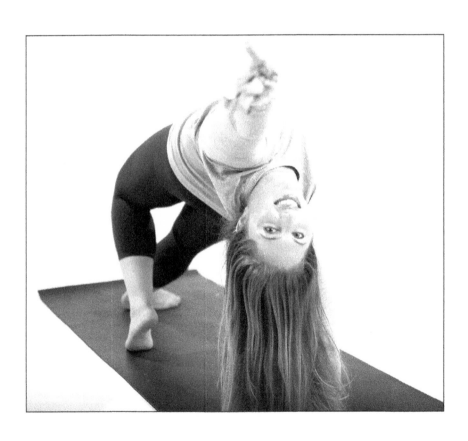

CHAPTER 8

WRITING TO THE DEPTHS

Context is everything.
—Lee Lozowick

For me, journal writing is one of the most valuable tools for transformation, and one that I consistently recommend to students and teachers alike. The context of my journaling process is for a deeper dive into self-knowledge and self-acceptance. For the purposes of this book, I invite you to join me in writing beyond body image, which is what we're all about here.

As we step out a bit from the shore, it is worth pointing out what journal writing is not, especially because so many have a negative view of themselves ("I can't write"; "What do *I* have to write about?"; "Jill is such a great writer, but I could never...") or because we fear our writing will be used against us in some way. In a recent course I taught, one of my students told me a former lover found her journal and read it, uninvited. She went on to share that she has never felt safe to write freely since that betrayal. After she shared her story, several other course participants told similar ones about how the privacy and sanctity of their journal or diary was violated. Moving beyond the pain of those past experiences is not easy . . . but writing can help in this endeavor and in many other challenges.

Writing Beyond Betrayal
AN EXERCISE

If you are dealing with a past betrayal or a violation of privacy with regard to your writing, write a letter to the people who invaded the sanctity of your work. (This exercise could also be used for any type of privacy violation or theft.) Tell them exactly what they did, how you felt then, how it has stayed with you, what it has cost you, and how you are no longer willing to be held down by the pain of their betrayal.

Read the letter out loud to yourself (or to a trusted friend) with some feeling, and several times.

Burn the letter. As you watch the pages burn, imagine the pain, the fear, the shame leaving you and making space for a new relationship with writing to emerge.

Many of us have had critical writing teachers, insensitive friends or nosy parents who disrespected our writing efforts. Many more of us have our own inner critic who won't quit. These wounds or self-defeating inner dialogues hamper creativity, self-expression and self-confidence to an alarming degree. Getting yourself out from under all the "shoulds" and "should nots" about writing to be able to use it as a tool for self-understanding requires some work, but is worthwhile. Again, writing can help in identifying and standing up to both inner and outer critics!

Challenging the Critics

AN EXERCISE

A thorough inventory in the form of a list is a good place to start dismantling some stuck energy around the wounds to your creativity and self-expression, without bogging you down with grammar, spelling or even the need to write long sentences. Here's how:

1. Make a list of some of the internal messages you have made up and accepted about your own writing. (For example, "Writing is hard for me.")
2. Choose one of those messages and write a list of defense points (reasons that support it). (Like, "It takes me forever to write a short letter.")
3. Choose the same message and write a list of prosecution points (reasons that challenge it). (For example, "Good writing takes time.")
4. Make a list of some ways you were hurt and discouraged in writing by the criticism or lack of acknowledgment of other people. List the person responsible for each incident of criticism or ignorance and add a few words to describe what happened.

Complete this exercise by reading back carefully over what you've written. Take three minutes (or more, as you wish) and write a few sentences in response to this prompt:

As a result of this writing exercise, I . . .

The Context of Curiosity

A context is like a frame around a picture that can determine the size and content of what can go inside. Generally, you wouldn't put a frame of neon lights around a priceless old masterpiece, for example. A context is also a defining purpose for some action: like your reason for a trip to Las Vegas might be to gamble, or to explore interesting architecture, or to eat great food. Where you go and what you do there would be determined by your context.

While some folks write for money, and we all write to communicate with distant friends, a most useful context for journal writing is to be curious about the hidden gems of knowledge that might live inside you. A context like this is quite challenging because it requires you to be courageous enough to explore what you may not already know about, both pleasant and unpleasant. C. Day-Lewis noted this theme (in *The Poetic Image*) many years ago. He said, "We do not write in order to be understood; we write in order to understand."[2] Inviting us a step further, contemporary author and writing teacher Natalie Goldberg (in *Writing Down the Bones*) suggested: "Write what disturbs you, what you fear, what you have not been willing to speak about. Be willing to be split open."[3]

Such curiosity- or self-knowledge writing is not about:

- getting the right answer or avoiding the wrong answer
- proper grammar, spelling, syntax
- sharing with others right away
- competition
- judgment
- achievement

---

[2]   Day-Lewis, C., (2006) *The Poetic Image,* Hong Kong: Hesperides Press.

[3]   Goldberg, Natalie. (1986) *Writing Down the Bones: Freeing the Writer Within.* Boulder, Colorado: Shambhala Publications.

- pleasing someone else
- publishing
- or any other externally referenced or internally critical reason.

Curiosity, not completeness. Exploration, not perfection. Courage, not correctness. Honesty, not praise. These are some of the virtues of writing to the depths.

What Context Are You In?

AN EXERCISE

Write down in stream-of-consciousness style or in list form:

1. What context or contexts would you ideally *like* to work from?

2. What context or contexts for life in general and your practice-life in particular would be most beneficial for you to hold?

3. Having considered what might be an optimal context, what is in your way of working toward or with that context? For instance: perfectionism, past wounds, disinterest, fear, time management, etc.

4. Choose one of these obstacles and write in greater depth about it for ten minutes:
   What holds me back from the ideal is …

5. Read slowly what you have written. Respond in writing to this prompt:
   As a result of this exercise I …

In Sutra 1:20 of the *Yoga Sutra*, Patanjali outlines five aspects to the path of yoga practice that are particularly relevant and applicable to our subject of self-understanding and self-acceptance:

1. Faithful certainty in the path (*shraddha*)
2. Directing energy towards the practices (*virya*)
3. Repeated memory of the path and the process of stilling the mind (*smirti*)
4. Training in deep concentration (*samadhi*), and
5. The pursuit of real knowledge, by which the higher samadhi is attained (*prajna*).

In the following section, I will take each of these five and relate it to life and yoga practice in general, and the practice of journal writing in particular.

Shraddha

Shraddha means faith. For our purposes here in considering the practice of journal writing, shraddha will not imply something religious . . . nor need it be overtly spiritual. In any type of activity, we need enough faith in the practice to get started and to engage the process. Here, I suggest we simply need faith in the practice of writing itself. We need some small belief or conviction that the process of writing will bear some kind of beneficial fruit.

Maybe you have tried writing in the past and without success, and memories are hampering your capacity to get going. Maybe you think you are not a writer. But, maybe you have a friend who loves to write and this relationship may be a touchstone or entry point for you: Although you do not have faith in the practice of writing for yourself, you have some faith in how much writing has helped him or her sort through difficulty. Even *faith in someone else's faith* in writing is a starting place.

In the New Testament, Jesus instructs his disciples that if they have faith the size of a mustard seed, they will be able to move mountains

(Matthew 17:20). I find this teaching extraordinarily helpful for work in all dimensions of life, and immediately applicable to journal writing. Faith need not be absolute, total or unwavering to be useful . . . no matter what we are attempting. We can proceed *with* doubt, misgivings and issues galore, so long as we have enough faith to take the first step and keep on stepping. With even a small seed of courage or persistence or intention as a place from which to start, so long as we do start, we can move mountains.

Whether or not the practice of writing or any practice will benefit us can only be determined after we give the endeavor a go for a while, which is why faith is important. No matter how inspired we may feel about starting, there are no guarantees. So, inherent in the faith we are speaking about is a kind of risk. Like so many practices in yogic life, despite our best efforts something might not "work," or work differently than we expected. For example, how many times have you wanted to sit in meditation to feel calmer only to meet your anger, restlessness or anxiety? How often have you gone to yoga class hoping for a bit of "time-out" only to meet your own self-criticism or insecurities? No matter how high our intentions are for ourselves, practice contains great unknowns and is not entirely predictable. We need some kind of daring faith to have the courage to begin.

Virya

Virya is the power of enthusiasm to make efforts. Virya may not equate to total conviction or complete resolution as much as the dedication required to make consistent efforts. As simple as it sounds, journal writing works best when we, *well* . . . actually write. And when, like any practice, we do it regularly. Obviously, we are busy people and not everyone will engage writing as a primary disciplined practice. Still, as with most practices, the small amounts we do are more beneficial than the large amounts we fail to do. Regularity and consistency create a time and place for the inner wisdom, creativity and spirit (sometimes referred to as "the Muse") to speak to you. Virya, in terms of a writing practice, may be less about overt enthusiasm and more about disciplined regularity.

In *The Haunted Heart: The Life and Times of Stephen King*, author Lisa Rogak recounts some of King's comments about his writing schedule: "There are certain things I do if I sit down to write," he said. "I have a glass of water or a cup of tea. There's a certain time I sit down, from 8:00 to 8:30, somewhere within that half hour every morning," he explained. "I have my vitamin pill and my music, sit in the same seat, and the papers are all arranged in the same places. The cumulative purpose of doing these things the same way every day seems to be a way of saying to the mind, 'You're going to be dreaming soon.'"[4]

Consistency and regularity require great will power to be sustained over time. Take care to consider the amount of energy sustainable for you. If your efforts are realistic, they will be doable, and your zeal can be maintained over the long haul.

Smriti

Smriti is cultivating a constant mindfulness of treading the path and of remembering the steps along the way. I think of smriti as "remembering to remember" the benefits of practice. Most of us know this with respect to asana. On plenty of days we do not want to practice and have to remind ourselves, "You always feel better after," or "Last time you felt this way, asana really helped clear your mind." Such reminders keep us in relationship with our intentions for practice. In terms of journal writing, smriti might express itself as remembering that, "Your journal is for you," or that, "There is no wrong or right way," and particularly, "There is wisdom inside that wants to express itself," and so on.

---

[4] Rogak, Lisa. (2008) *The Haunted Heart: The Life and Times of Stephen King.* New York: St. Martin's Press.

No matter how clear our intention, how disciplined and enthusiastic our efforts are, there will be times when we do not want to practice. Resistance is part of the process of practice, not a sign something is wrong with the practice or with us. When we feel resistant to writing, the resistance itself is a great subject to write about. Smriti is how we remember not only our reasons for practice but also the techniques of practice so that our intellectual training can bolster our waxing and waning willpower.

Samadhi

Oddly, unless we are in a meditation class or engaged in sutra study, we rarely talk about *samadhi*. In the average asana practice or in most yoga forums, samadhi isn't considered. Nonetheless, let's engage samadhi here and apply it to writing practice!

Without a huge philosophical discourse, we might simply consider samadhi as the "stilling" or the "cessation of the identifications with the fluctuations of the mind." In terms of writing, samadhi will help us in two primary ways:

1. When we write regularly, we can learn to observe patterns of thought and patterns of feeling characterizing the process for us. Initially, this type of self-observation runs the risk of becoming more like rumination or self-obsession. Many people actually get stuck in this stage of journal writing and quit. It's no wonder. How boring and redundant to keep writing endlessly of your same old fears, projections, feelings of inadequacy, etc. Over time, however, another possibility can emerge with journal writing—a possibility similar to what happens in a meditation practice. We start to experience a certain distance from the content of the writing, which allows us some space. We get to see the thoughts and feelings for what they are: just thoughts and feelings—not the whole truth and not requiring immediate action or compulsive avoidance, but

simply the movements of the mind. This clarity allows for a small measure of dis-identification with the thoughts, or a samadhi-like moment of reprieve from the incessant narrative of our mind stream.

This dis-identifying process lies at the heart of moving deeper than body image. So much of the painful obsession with appearance happens because we are *believing* everything we think about how we look or how we should look. Learning to observe those thoughts without believing them, needing to act on them, or needing to compulsively avoid them is the essence of meditation and the essence of moving beyond body image.

2. The root of samadhi is "same" or "even," implying a sameness or evenness in consciousness. Also, the word implies a "putting together in the same place." And so, while this idea is not exactly the meditative consciousness Patanjali was outlining, we can use journal writing to bring together various voices and messages living within our minds and hearts and allow them expression. In so doing, we allow ourselves an experience of wholeness because we are, "putting ourselves together in the same place."

Prajna

Prajna is the higher wisdom that comes from discrimination, and this wisdom is assiduously sought through the process of introspection. In a sense, this faculty is the overarching context of accessing our inner wisdom. Stephen King wrote, "Writing is refined thinking." Writing, in this sense, is the process of refining our thinking, clarifying our wisdom and articulating our truth.

Opportunities to abandon our own inner wisdom abound in the culture at large, as well as in yoga culture. For anyone needing help navigating the current world of "fake news" and manipulative political tactics, as well as for yoga practitioners who want to grow on the path without being coerced, converted or convinced into believing something they may not hold to be true, writing is one of the best tools for holding fast to our own inner knowing. Writing is a useful way to integrate experience with inner understanding so that wisdom truly dawns.

About the Five Aspects

AN EXERCISE

1. Pick one of the five aspects discussed in the previous section—faith, memory, enthusiasm, samadhi, wisdom—and write about why it caught your attention now.

2. Respond in writing to the following: *How can your yoga practice help you understand writing as a practice? In what ways are they similar? In what ways are they different?*

Morning Pages

From Julia Cameron, author of *The Artist's Way*:

> Morning Pages are three pages of longhand, stream-of-consciousness writing, done first thing in the morning. There is no wrong way to do Morning Pages—they are not high art. They are not even "writing." They are about anything and everything that crosses your mind—and they are for your eyes only. Morning Pages provoke, clarify, comfort, cajole, prioritize and synchronize the day at hand. Do not over-think Morning Pages: just put three pages of anything on the page . . . and then do three more pages tomorrow.

In her work, Julia Cameron outlines two main tenets of the practice of Morning Pages: Do them first thing in the morning and write in longhand for three pages. I feel obligated to suggest that, as modern householder-yogis, these simple constraints may not be doable. Maybe "first thing in the morning" for you is filled with crying infants, a mate who needs your help or a dog that needs walking. If you can manage the exact protocol, great. However, one shouldn't let the "perfect" get in the way of the "good-enough."

If you can do one page of writing after your kids get to school, that is wonderful. Or perhaps, you have a break between classes or teaching private lessons where you can scribble out two pages. That too is awesome. Perhaps setting a timer will work better for you and you can write for five minutes. Variations on the theme are endless. Regular practice of any kind is better than the perfect protocol that you do not do.

In fact, "Don't let the perfect get in the way of the good-enough" is my motto for just about every kind of practice or protocol—from meditation to asana to pranayama to mantra to diet and so on. Something is almost always better than nothing. We must not let our perfectionistic tendencies rob of us of the joy of turning inward through practice. A little practice goes a long way, and we need to validate whatever efforts we make, large or small.

Another helpful hint is just to "keep your hand moving" on the page (as Natalie Goldberg recommends) even if you all you write is, "I can't think of anything to say; this is so stupid; I hate this . . ." The act of moving your hand on the page will activate your brain and is one of the best ways to move beyond typical writer's block. This action-based approach is just like asana practice. So often, when we do not feel like practicing, if we can just do one downward-facing-dog pose, our mind will start to get interested in the posture. It is easier to get interested in the posture from the posture than from the sofa or chair.

The context for Morning Pages is quite reminiscent of the context for meditation. This type of journal writing is not about getting anywhere or trying to figure anything out. We are not attempting to be positive or insightful. We simply enter the stream of our mind consciously and give it expression. Much like meditation, what can happen is an unfolding of a different relationship to our thoughts, their patterns and movements, as well as a keener understanding of the voices of wisdom that also live in the midst of the roiling of thought.

Morning Pages
AN EXERCISE

- Practice Morning Pages NOW. Use a timer to give yourself a time limit, like 10 minutes, or aim for 1-3 pages; and keep your hand moving the whole time!
- Daily, for at least this next week, add Morning Pages to your practice routine, giving yourself the chance to evaluate its usefulness.

Symbols

For many of us, our intellectual and rational mind stands as a guardian at the gate of our inner wisdom. Many of us like things in our lives to make sense, to confirm and conform to our already existing understanding of ourselves and the world, and to function within boundaries of rational thought. There is no fundamental problem with a rational orientation to life. People with a highly developed sense of the rational often make sane life choices and can make useful distinctions professionally, personally and relationally. They tend to be good at planning, accomplishing and making progress throughout their lives. *All hail to the highly competent rational thinkers in our midst!*

However, when we limit our inner lives to the rational worldview of our intellectual self, we miss out on the wide world of possibilities existing in what I refer to as "non-rational." Different than "irrational," the non-rational aspect of who we are may not make immediate, linear sense to ourselves or the rest of the world, but is highly intuitive, insightful, feeling-based, spiritually-connected and at peace with paradoxes, co-exiting truths and our authentic wisdom.

Symbols are another tool that, used with writing, might allow you to bypass the rational guardian aspect of intellect and invite a different kind of inner knowing to surface. For most of us, when we hear the word "dog" what we see is not the word itself but an inner image of a dog. Maybe I see Locket and you see Snoopy, and someone else sees their stuffed-animal dog from childhood. The point is that we are wired to relate to language and words through image and impressions because the English language itself is a representation of something, not the thing itself.

This phenomenon is particularly true with the deep levels of the psyche that function more symbolically and non-rationally than do our waking, ordinary, participatory selves. Think about how dreams function. The dream-self cooks up a bunch of images, which rarely make a lot of sense but can be de-coded over time to provide a wealth of knowledge about our own growth and evolution. Icons from spiritual traditions are also symbolic, encoded with meaning that can seep into our consciousness beyond the rational level of the mind. Of course, this idea is not so far out or mystical, if you think about it—marketing agencies use this unconscious symbolic access all the time to influence how we think, feel and spend.

Working with symbols can be applied to any domain of your process to gain insight and clarity, and to invite a broader perspective and way of knowing. For instance, you might look for a small object in nature speaking beauty to you. Or look around your house for an object that represents wholeness.

Once again, the context is curiosity and affirming you have answers inside that you can learn to access, learn from and take guidance from.

Eventually, this type of self-inquiry will become more familiar and even enjoyable.

Symbols and Writing
SUGGESTIONS FOR PRACTICE

1. Look around your surroundings—your home, your office, the studio, or wherever you find yourself today. Ask your Inner Wisdom to show you a symbol that represents your connection to the source of your inner strength. It might be a flower, an icon on your personal shrine or altar, a mala, a picture, etc. Don't over-think it, and trust whatever feels right.
2. Take the symbol and place it in front of you.
3. Describe the symbol physically, use writing.
4. Write about how the object you found (or that found you) symbolizes your connection to the source of your inner strength.
5. Imagine the symbol has its own voice and let it speak to you about what it is, what it knows, and what it has to teach you.
6. Underline any recurring words and/or statements, any insights that stand out for any reason in what you have written.
8. Write for a few minutes about your experience of this process:
   As a result of this writing I . . .

PART IV

TEACHING AND BEING YOGA

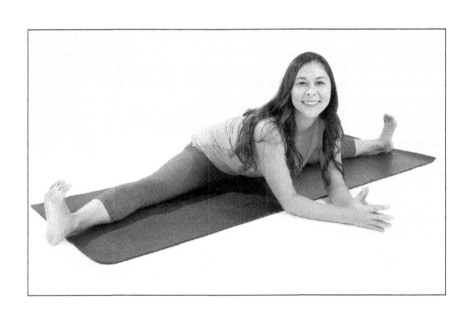

CHAPTER 9

THE 4-FOLD EDUCATIONAL PROCESS OF YOGA

Yoga is an educational process requiring inspiration, information, direct experience and integration. As these processes come alive within the practitioner, the practices and principles of yoga provide a true sense of sanctuary and shelter. And, although the average public yoga class or teacher-training program may not speak directly to these four aspects of learning, I see these stages embedded into the fabric of yoga.

From relaxing to working out, from the use of Sanskrit chants to rock 'n roll playlists, from fluid flows to static postures, the diversity of yoga presentation today increases. The economic impact of yoga and its associated products and services is also on the rise, creating a culture of competitive, distracting and even disheartening consumerism. Because of these inherent challenges, I want to outline and describe yoga as an educational process to make a clear distinction between an educational and a consumer-oriented context for yoga.

I understand we live in a capitalistic country and yoga studios, and you as teachers, are often struggling to make ends meet. Additionally, many of your students have trouble accessing classes and trainings due to increased costs of living and other socio-economic variables. On every step of study, obstacles and difficulties dwell. With the proliferations of studios—both online and in person—we may not have to climb to the mountain top to find a "yoga-guru" anymore. But the process of learning, overall, may not be any easier or more straightforward than in the past. Seeing the endeavor as educational can be more useful than expecting it to conform to consumer-oriented standards.

Practice What You Love

In general, I think people should practice the yoga they enjoy. Like to move? You will probably be more at home with *vinyasa*. Like the heat? Go to the hot studio. Like details? Find a good alignment teacher. While a case can be made for expanding beyond an initial attraction or avoidance, my general observation is that students and teachers will have the best success with practices they actually enjoy. And, in the twenty years I have been teaching asana, I've found that, regardless of entry point—alignment, flow, quiet, loud, etc.—students who stay committed to practice for over five years will expand beyond their initial patterns naturally . . . in their own time, for their own reasons: Sometimes injuries make alignment more relevant; sometimes personal losses bring the need for meditation and philosophical inquiry. It all depends. However, if we stay the course and continue with the practice, we will realize what we have been paying our hard-earned money and spending our precious time to accomplish.

The process of learning will be as unsettling as comforting: While we may want freedom from our negative mental chatter, we may find ourselves instead facing a roiling mind for an entire class or practice session. We may want to feel good about ourselves but find negative comparisons with others—in terms of looks, ability, knowledge— dominate our attention every time we practice. We may want a meaningful relationship with our teacher or community, but find ourselves feeling left out, unacknowledged or misunderstood. Sooner or later, the very thing we came to yoga to get free of will show up in our life of practice.

From a consumer-oriented viewpoint, this state of affairs will seem like something is going wrong. We think, "I did not come here to feel left out. I have felt left out my whole life!" From an educational viewpoint, however, landing in the middle of our psychological patterns is not necessarily bad news. If we aim at drawing forth our inner wisdom, then we will also be drawing forth those aspects of who we are that stand in the way of that wisdom. As the saying goes, "You can't heal it, if you don't feel it." In order to move beyond our limited conditioning, we often have to get to know our conditioned patterns very well.

The educational perspective is not intended to excuse abuse or psychologically negligent behavior on the part of our teachers, or to minimize feelings of betrayal or disappointment that are natural in long-term teacher-student dynamics. Rather, this perspective is intended as an empowering context diminishing perfectionistic expectations of yourself and others while increasing patience and compassion in your life of practice and learning.

The Four Aspects of the Educational Process of Yoga

1. Inspiration and Aim
2. Information and Theory
3. Practice and Experience
4. Articulation and Integration

Inspiration and Aim

Inspiration is the doorway into the realm of feeling. For some, the feeling realm is emotionally oriented, involving human sentiments, and personal narratives and meanings. For others, a less-personal, more universal sense of mood, or *bhava*, longing and devotion anchors the feeling realm.

Emotions often stand guard in protecting the less rational aspects of our being, such as intuition and instinct. While personal emotions are not always valued in traditional yoga teachings, I believe that the free-flow of emotions—where feelings are neither ignored nor dramatized but are given expression in and through the body with mindful awareness—is necessary. Such flow provides the internal barometer necessary for discernment of right and wrong, along with spiritual wisdom. With a full range of feelings, we can use anger to alert us when our boundaries and needs are not met. We can use grief as an authentic response to loss, and fear to remind us of our limits. We will have joy to express love and delight, and to infuse our lives with lighthearted acceptance.

We cannot expect to reliably access our inner wisdom and spiritual inspiration if we stifle authentic emotions or over-react based on past impressions. We don't need to be perfect, without vices, or completely free of conditioned patterns to taste the nectar of inspiration and wisdom. However, an ever-maturing relationship to our feelings and mood will deepen our ability to trust our instincts and intuition.

Inspiration in the educational process is not about preaching or lecturing. Education (from *educare*) is a "drawing forth" from within, not a process of converting, persuading or coercing ourselves with dogma or doctrine. Inspiration speaks to the heart and spirit of our work as students and teachers, and helps answer the WHY of the practice: *Why should any of us engage the difficulties inherent in a path requiring awareness, honesty, discipline and dedication?*

In troubled times, heart-opening practices can be even more troubling—as the heart opens, we feel *more* and we do not always feel *better*. A heart-opening path such as yoga may not always soothe the spirit in troubling times because the path may bring us closer to the heart of the trouble itself—suffering. Living with an open heart in the midst of fires, floods, famines, oppression and abuse is not easy. This difficult situation is exactly where we find ourselves as modern yoga practitioners and teachers.

There is no single reason why anyone practices (or teaches) yoga. Some people need a "time out" from the stresses of their family, their job, their habitual modes of being and behaving. Some people look for a way to work *out*. Some are looking for a way to work *in*.

What is common is that each of us has his or her own reasons; what is essential is that we practice and stay closely connected to our own aims and intentions. Aim is absolutely vital for longevity on the path, especially during troubled times.

The Inspiration and Aim stage of learning links us up to the power of the breath and the power of Spirit—to what *animates* each of us. Whether our intention and inspiration for practice are expressed in overtly spiritual language or not, generally a thread connects even the most materially-based intention to something more heart-oriented and spiritual. For instance, someone who wants to lose weight often wants to improve health or simply appearance. But as health improves, well-being often improves, self-confidence increases, discipline and awareness are built—all of which translate into qualities far from the superficial in our lives.

Suggestions for Writing Practice

1. What inspires you?
2. As a lifelong student, what do your teachers do that you find inspiring?
3. What seems to inspire your students?
4. What do these observations (1–3) tell you about your own experience and capacity to inspire?

Information and Theory

While we need inspiration to get on the path of learning, we also need tangible means by which to do the work. We need information— books, teachers, instructions—if we want to learn asana. Otherwise, our inspiration will be thwarted.

The Information aspect of yoga ranges from anatomy and movement principles, to philosophical study, to contemplation techniques. Whether we teach others or not, a good grasp on sequencing methods, modifications and adaptations will serve us considerably. Both teachers and students benefit from functional interpersonal skills, and our increasingly troubled times now demand that we navigate a dynamic and disturbing social, political and cultural landscape. (If you feel overwhelmed, or long for the days where a good sequence and a little yoga philosophy was enough to aid you in your yoga journey, you are not alone.)

The Information stage of learning has huge applications to personal growth and development outside the classroom or formal practice arenas. Knowing even a little about the road map for recovery from addiction or trauma, knowing what fosters healthy relationships, keeping up-to-date on trends and jobs, and deepening our own study of spirituality are invaluable in navigating the inevitable problems and questions that arise for us, and supporting our students in ways and means to support themselves. And as with Information, a knowledge of Theory about the life of practice helps us in meeting the necessary challenges that will come our way.

Information and Theory together are like the big X–YOU ARE HERE spot on a map—they can help you get your bearings in life, teaching and practice, which can alleviate stress, worry and isolation, and take some of the guesswork out of the process.

As yoga practitioners and teachers in troubled times, we may long to create shelter from the storms of life in our own practice and that of our students, but not know how. I suggest we can turn our thinking minds to the optimal context for practice and begin a brainstorming process of what attributes and skills will bring that context to life. If yoga is, as I assert, a process of drawing wisdom forth from within, we need our guides and teachers to provide us with information about how to use the practice to access our inner resources.

The 4-Fold Educational Process of Yoga

As teachers, no matter how sincere, talented, experienced and well-trained we are, if we attempt to bolster others from the outside-in, we will eventually burn out from the sheer impossibility of holding so much responsibility for others. What we can hope to do is point people to their interior sources of refuge and shelter through practice. As teachers, our job is to deliver our students to the practices so that the practice can deliver our students to the shelter within themselves.

What might this mean for an average class? As teachers, a practical application of the Information stage of learning is to be direct and clear about what you are doing and why. Whether that is to say, "This is why we use a block for *trikonasana,*" or to offer a lengthier explanation about the value of visualization techniques, we give people information so they are intelligently informed about the process they are engaging. For example, I might say:

> Today we are going to do a visualization to contact a source of inner strength. Visualization requires attention and imagination, and for some of you the imagination aspect may lack concrete facts and even create cynicism. What we are after in a visualization is to feel strength from within. I could simply tell you that you are strong, but if you feel such strength from within, the experience itself will be empowering. The process is simple. I will ask you to close your eyes, guide you to your breath, and then give you some cues to go inward and imagine an inner sanctuary. If you are "super rational," just suspend a little of that for today and see what you get.

While the exact wording may vary from teacher to teacher, and from time to time, the gist of what I am describing remains the same—we empower the student's innate wisdom. I do this kind of preparatory explanation throughout my classes, workshops and trainings. Educating the intellect is different from jumping straight into the experience and using bold assertions such as, "We all have an inner sanctuary. I will lead you there." Educating the intellect gives sane, clear, outlines for the *how* and *why* of practice, and allows each student to enter the process as informed and responsible as possible, given the parameters and limits of various learning environments. For instance, a 60-minute public asana class may not allow enough time for in-depth explanations about every verbal cue or teaching point. Yet, it is still possible to create an informed and consensual educational environment.

For students, the Information stage comes alive when they take responsibility for their learning process by reading, studying, asking questions and exploring the concepts for themselves over time. When we are continuing our own training, it is important for us to do the same. If another teacher or trainer offers a technique that does not make sense to us after we try it, we can empower ourselves to ask questions for greater clarity and understanding. If our teachers cannot explain why they are teaching this technique, we should consider looking for additional resources and helpers to assist us in deepening our knowledge. We can encourage our students to do the same with us, and with others. No one teacher can have all of the answers anyone might need over the life of practice, and as we develop our understanding through study and practice, our needs and interests are likely to shift and change.

The Information stage of the educational process is one of the best remedies for destructive psychological dynamics between teachers and students. Strong, clear information-sharing helps dismantle blind trust, magical thinking, and the tendencies to seek validation and approval from an outer charismatic leader. When we, as students or teachers, become empowered participants in the process of practice—which is nothing other than the process of coming into relationship with our own wisdom—we will be less easily manipulated, coerced or overpowered by the shadow elements invariably existing in outside authorities. Information and theory are no guarantee these difficulties will not arise, but "empowered studentship" is one of the best ways to safeguard our own authority in the process of learning from others.

Suggestions for Writing Practice

1. Have you ever been "thrown into" a learning environment without explanation in a way that was beneficial? What happened? What was the positive outcome of jumping into experience without information?

2. Have you ever been "thrown into" a learning environment without explanation in a way that was damaging, painful, upsetting? What happened? What were the negative repercussions to jumping into experience without information?

3. When has Theory helped you as a student or teacher in the classroom or in your life outside of the classroom?

4. When has having Theory been a hindrance?

Practice and Experience

The four aspects of the yoga learning process are not discreet or separate from one another. In fact, they have plenty of overlap. Inspiration (and feeling) meets and relates to Information (and the intellect), and both serve the unfolding of the Practice itself through Experience, which can only happen through action. The action may be visualization or meditation, involving a more inward turning of attention; or the action may be more outward such as asana, writing or chanting. Regardless of expression, the Experience aspect of the learning process is "the practice of the practice" as opposed to the theory of the practice or the inspiration behind the practice.

As teachers, the Experience component is the difference between sermonizing or lecturing and facilitating an expression or action that will deliver the student to their internal connection to shelter, refuge, strength and hope. As students, the Experience component is where we take the journey our teachers have been outlining and where we come into a direct knowing that is personal and authentic. As important as context and information are to the process of learning, the Practice itself generally holds the power for transformation. Inspiration and Information are necessary, but until the teachings are internalized and realized through ongoing practice, we will still be encouraging reliance on outside testimony rather than direct knowledge. As simple as the analogy might sound, the Experience stage moves us from descriptions of sugar or honey to the taste of sweetness itself.

Of course, practice is not always "sweet" along the way. One of my former yoga teachers used to work a lot with timed poses in the early days of my study with him. He would take us through standing-pose sequences with one-minute timings for each posture. Timed poses require mental dedication and physical effort. Inspired by what he taught at his workshops, I started using timings in my home practice. I set the timer for one minute and found that, without his cues and the group energy to lean on, I could not stay more than fifteen seconds in the pose without feeling agitated and frustrated. Over time, I realized it was not my body that was tired, but that my attention was not trained for the long holds without the outer support of the teacher and the class. I kept working at the timings, however, and eventually the one-minute holds were no problem at all.

Many years later, when I was struggling in my marriage, I talked to this same yoga teacher about how I was working through the difficulty. When I said, "Well, it's like the timed poses you used to teach." He looked at me questioningly. "The thing about timings is that my mind always wants to get out of the pose before my body is actually at its limit," I told him. "The timings taught me that the desire to 'get out' has many levels, so I have been practicing staying and working in my marriage like it is a pose, rather than getting out just because I want to. The only way to stay a minute or more in a pose is to keep my mind busy on the work of the pose, not focused on the desire to get out. So like that."

He nodded with understanding.

The irony about this story is that this particular teacher wasn't oriented toward monogamy. And yet, the practice he taught helped me maintain my own vows. I think of this as a great example of how yoga teachers can teach people to practice, and practice can teach people how to live. But if yoga teachers try to teach people how to live, then chances are the teachers have crossed the line from educating and inspiring into preaching, sermonizing, converting and/or coercing.

Of course, sometimes we as teachers can help our students to connect the dots from experience within the practice to application in life outside. In my story, my sustained practice, not my teacher's commentaries or his own life example, gave me a reference point for how to be challenged and still remain in place.

Whether the turbulence we face is personal (like my marriage at the time), or cultural (like so much of what is happening in the political landscape today), the peace we are seeking comes from the source to which practice is pointing us. And, to get the fruits of practice … well, we have to do the practice!

Our teaching in troubled times gets tricky. Are we acknowledging the difficulties that all humans are facing, so as not to turn the yoga classroom into an ivory-tower environment where suffering is ignored? Can we do this without giving so much detail and personal opinion that we intrude on the individual inquiry and self-examination yoga can provide? While no cliché or any single formula will assure this delicate balance, a few carefully considered words can go a long way. Here are some that I've used and found useful:

1. "I don't know about you, but one tour through my newsfeed this morning and I was broken-hearted."

2. "Regardless of what side of the political aisle you sit on, very few of us are here today for more division, more judgment or more bad news."

3. "So, we are clear, the assurances of 'it's all good' that yoga offers, refer to something much deeper than politics, Congress's tax bill, and whatever tragedy is in today's news cycle. The deep assurances of yoga are hard to feel in the midst of modern times and they do not necessarily take away our human heart-felt concerns."

4. "I am glad we are all here together today. Clearly, we are at a time in history where racial tensions are high, where misunderstandings hit deep, and where fear is close to the surface. Yoga won't make any of that go away, but for this hour, we can move, breathe and shift our focus in such a way we might grow strong enough to keep our hearts open in the face of what we are all experiencing."

Chances are, each of these sentences might have its own problems, and therefore may not be workable for you. Some acknowledgement can be useful; too much acknowledgement can be its own kind of problem. My experience is that while no one wants or needs a lecture when they come to class, many people are coming to our classes feeling beaten up by current events and trends. And while "the practice of the practice" will deliver folks to a certain sort of solution, many people won't feel safe or validated enough to take the journey of practice without an intelligent acknowledgement of the difficult starting point.

We can encourage our students to be discriminating in where they invest their trust regarding teachers and teachings. If, as a student (and even the most highly experienced among us will continue our training), your teacher makes an effort to acknowledge certain difficulties and his or her message does not resonate for you, perhaps you can examine your own reaction more closely to determine what course of action to take in relationship to your teacher. Yoga teachers, for all our great traits and training, have blind spots, unexamined biases and unchecked prejudices that can be enormous and problematic. Sometimes, those problem areas, when honestly discussed, can open the doors to greater understanding and intimacy between you and your teacher. Sometimes, open dialogue is not possible. I have been in plenty of classes and trainings where I didn't agree with everything the teacher said and could still benefit from the learning environment. I have also been in situations which, upon close examination, were toxic and ceased being useful for me. There is no formula for navigating the process I am describing.

Remember, our teachers are there to help us learn to practice so that inner wisdom comes forth from within, not to entertain us, agree with us, or to confirm our ideas and/or biases. Only you can decide for yourself what is workable for you.

Integration and Articulation

As we approach this fourth domain, Integration and Articulation, I recall that my spiritual teacher always said the degree to which we were able to *articulate* our learning was the degree to which we had *integrated* it into our lives. When we have been inspired, informed and had a direct encounter with the teaching through practice, and when we can *then explain* the learning clearly to someone else, we know wisdom has truly been drawn forth from within.

One of my friends has a son in a charter school focused on experiential learning. Her son and I were discussing the non-traditional evaluation system used at his school. He said that for every lesson he fills out a form with one of three options from which to choose:

1. I do not understand the lesson.
2. I understand the lesson.

3. I could explain the lesson to someone else.

The Integration and Articulation stage of the learning process falls under the third option. Keep in mind that not all forms of articulation are the same. Some of us are highly verbal—we will articulate our learning readily in words, either spoken or written. Some of us are visual and may paint a picture. We may also express our understanding more kinesthetically, articulating an action in our bodies in asana, or through our actions in life, without keen capacity to describe exactly what is going on. All that being said, the Articulation/Integration stage tends to preference the verbal learners a bit. But for those of you who may have super-powers in other areas, do not worry—there is more than one way!

Yoga was originally an oral tradition. Much of the teaching has been passed down through the ages by speaking and listening to verbal language, to words. Even the great sages were reported to have "heard" the teachings. But the rishis were the "Seers—they *saw* something beyond normal sight.

In a yoga class, most likely our teacher instructs us through a series of poses with teaching methods leaning heavily on verbal cues. Props, hands-on adjustments, partner work and demonstrations support the verbal mode, while adding kinesthetic and visual tools. As students, we are expected to take mostly verbal cues and translate them into action with awareness (sensory/kinesthetic) in the body. When we teach, we have to take the various processes we accessed as students and articulate our understanding in the best way we can to guide someone else to their own experience.

Personally, I suspect that yoga teaching often goes awry because so many teachers try to teach concepts and poses that have not yet been fully integrated within themselves. A teacher's capacity to articulate the ideas or techniques therefore is limited. Even in philosophical studies, we will powerfully communicate to others only something we have studied well; and better yet, when we have experienced and integrated the teaching for ourselves. For example, when someone with many years of meditation talks about "a unified field of energy," you can actually *feel* the reality of the field they are speaking about. A brand-new teacher saying the same words might sound fluffy or even confused.

Despite the challenges, to teach is a great gift to us as practitioners. The articulation required to instruct others helps us clarify what we *do not* know, improve our understanding of what we *do* know, and gives us opportunities to realize what we knew but *didn't know* that we knew. Commonly, I've said something in class that surprised me, something that unexpectedly came through from my own wisdom. Sometimes, inspirational messages come pouring forth with great insight and clarity; at other times, I recognize (and can share) an alignment connection, on the spot, as I teach.

As teachers, one practical way we can assist students in articulating their experience is to occasionally give them opportunities to voice their process. A few examples:

- Teach a pose in two different ways and then ask the group, "What did you notice? What was the difference in the two different approaches?"

  or

- When a student has a breakthrough, we can ask, "What made the difference?" This gives the student a chance to anchor their learning through articulation (*to know what they know*), and also gives us a chance to collect insight about which methods and cues are helpful for certain poses and certain types of students in poses.

  or

- When a student is struggling with a pose, ask them, "Can you articulate exactly what the issue is for you?"

As students, we can do this for ourselves in our personal practice and in class. When we have ease or challenge in a pose on a given day, the more we can ask ourselves "Why?" and, "Where do the differences lie?" the more we will be integrating our experience through the process of articulation.

Inspiration, knowledge and experience move into wisdom through integration and articulation. In troubling times, we are bombarded with information, misinformation and a cacophony of voices competing for our allegiance. We do not live in a time where the outside sources of information are always reliable or hold our best interests in mind. Learning to access, integrate and rely on our inner wisdom is not just an esoteric idea, but a survival strategy for times like these. Not simply a vague principle or a good idea, the capacity to trust ourselves is immensely practical and immediately relevant. Whether we want to avoid manipulative cult dynamics, coercive psychological tactics or simply manage our mood a little better when scrolling through Facebook, inner wisdom is key.

Suggestions for Practice

1. Articulate your learning: Identify one pose you were once unable to do that you are now able to do. Write about or speak to a friend about what was the initial problem or block with the pose? How did you overcome it? What specifically came together in your practice that made a once-undoable pose into a pose that you can now do?

2. Articulate your learning: Identify a situation in your personal or professional life in which you feel like you have experienced growth. Write down what your initial issue was. Write about how the issue manifested. What changed? What specifically shifted in this situation, inside yourself, etc., that allowed for your experience of growth?

Learning to access, trust and rely upon our inner wisdom is often easier said than done. Like any respectful and enduring relationship, this kind of intimacy with ourselves takes time. And, while the rewards are great, the lessons rarely come cheaply. Recognizing and acknowledging the difficulty and rewards of the learning process can help both teachers and students have compassion for one another, lower unrealistic expectations of the learning process itself, and discover a humble and clear foundation upon which to build.

—Christina Sell

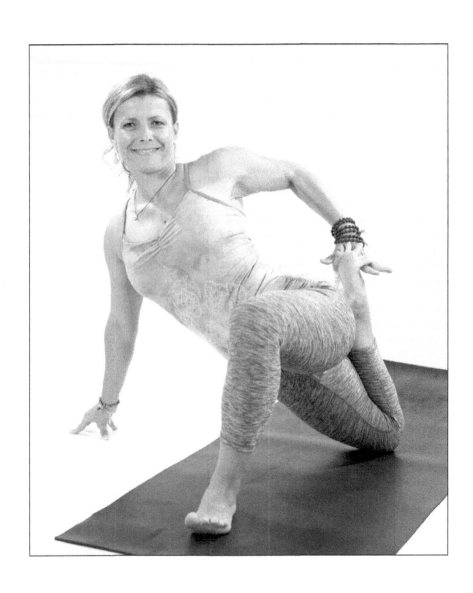

CHAPTER 10

ISSUES AND INSPIRATION FOR TEACHERS

I am interested in a vision of yoga that is not anchored in some utopian dream, but, is instead grounded in a paradigm of "good enough." Of course, depending on who we are, "good enough" can vary significantly, making the whole topic even more daunting to actualize reliably. For instance, for folks who come to yoga with a history of physical abuse, a class "good enough" not to re-injure and perhaps even provide a healing opportunity is likely very different than for someone who is not coping with trauma from those wounds. Same goes for those suffering issues with race, size, gender, socio-economic status, education, physical abilities and limitations, illness, health, addictions, etc. And yet, part of the unrealistic, utopian yoga dream (as I see it) is the expectation—conscious or unconscious—that one approach "fits all." That one class we offer or one set of cues we give or avoid giving can somehow address the myriad needs in any given community of practitioners.

I recently had a discussion with a colleague who outlined a vision for a yoga that was inclusive, politically active, trauma sensitive, egalitarian and more. I nearly had a panic attack hearing the description; no way could or would *my* public classes and workshops meet such a standard. Even if I were doing my best to reach the high bar she set (and to be clear, I try to do a good job), there would be people in my classrooms who, despite my best efforts, would eventually feel hurt, ignored, unseen, unable and left out. Some of this would be my fault due to my unconscious patterns and biases, and some would be due to theirs.

Certainly, there is always room for improvement and greater clarity. We probably need to do better as teachers and as an industry . . . and I am not discounting that reality. Issues abound, and I think naming problems for what they are is important for us to know where to apply our efforts toward improvement. Still, as time goes by, the less I have come to expect yoga to provide all and everything.

The asana practice has been a great form of awareness, physical expression and discipline for me. I also love to hike, bike and paddle a kayak. As much as I love asana, it does not satisfy me completely as my sole physical activity. And, while I have had few chronic injuries from asana, I also go to professional body-workers of all kinds to help with my aches, pains, unique tweaks and peculiarities. For instance, when my hip hurt, I had an MRI. What helped my pain the most was an injection of anti-inflammatories, not yoga therapy.

I have found immense psychological resources in the teachings and practices of yoga. I also have a great psychotherapist. I find some yoga philosophy enriching and inspiring. I also go to church, read across many spiritual disciplines, and right now I find more solace in contemplative prayer, time in nature, being with my dog and writing in my journal than I do in the average dharma talk, church service or yoga class.

Some of my favorite people are my yoga friends, students and colleagues. I have also found that having friends who don't care about "anything yoga" to be immensely valuable. These outliers oftentimes possess a practical unencumbered wisdom that can be hard to find in spiritual communities so often bogged down in rights and wrongs. I have profound gratitude for my yoga teachers, and yet I have found they are all human. They do not always see me in my best light, and they have each, at some point along the way, misjudged my motives or said hurtful things.

I don't teach asana because I think it is everything anyone needs for a happy, healthy meaningful life wrapped up in one package. Perhaps, because so much of my public life revolves around my work as a teacher, asana may appear elevated beyond what it is for me—an important facet of the diamond of my full life expression. As much as I've invested in asana and yogic philosophy over the years, their value in my life today exists more in how they have influenced all the other facets of my life, not in their singularity of expression. But let's face it, most of my readers know me because of yoga, not because I love my dog, I am a good cook, I help my father, I have a wicked sense of humor, I like alpine lakes, I have a great art collection and so on. The parts of my life that fill in the fullness of who I am are not as publicized as the backbends, arm balances and teacher trainings. And the fuller the other areas become for me, the more a yoga that is good enough is . . . *well*, good enough.

Lessons, Hard Won

Years ago, my primary yoga teacher at the time was facing criticism from the community as his work grew beyond a small group of students into a global network. His long-term students were missing the close personal connection they had with him in the early days; a familiarity that had served as the foundation of his expanding empire. Additionally, new students felt disconnected, unseen and invalidated because, in any given workshop, they were swimming unnoticed in a sea of people. What the "old-timers" reported about their early days with this teacher wasn't being felt by the new people. It was like the old "emperor" was naked, while most of the townsfolk were pretending otherwise . . . at first.

More could be (and has been) said about this teacher and that time. In my estimation, as the school grew in scale from a close-knit bonded group into a worldwide movement, the mechanisms of leadership failed to adapt effectively, leaving both old and new students hurt and frustrated.

At one conference, attempting to quell this rising tide of discontent, my teacher told the group how he was "there for everybody." I remember thinking to myself, "Oh, boy, we are in for it now. There is *no way* he can be there for everybody. The only way this can end is badly." Later that week, I begged him to change his narrative so that he stopped promising something he could not deliver.

I think he *wanted* to be there for everybody. And I think the scale of his experiment was no longer as satisfying *for him* either, without the deeper connections that marked the early days of his teaching work. Instead of making bigger, more impossible promises, I wanted him to talk honestly about his limitations and how a larger community cannot provide the same things as a small community can. As a yoga school, I wanted us to understand that, even with such limits, it was possible to have many of our needs met, but probably not all of them. I wanted us to acknowledge that a solid yogic education—one complete with spiritual inspiration and community connection—does not require perfection of the teacher, ourselves or one another.

Sadly, that shift in narrative did not happen.

Let me pause the story here to add a few side notes. Unlike some others, I personally did not feel abused or traumatized by my involvement with this teacher. He hurt my feelings, for sure. I hurt his feelings in return. We had fights. We had misunderstandings and differing views. I made choices he probably still sees as betrayal. And, a lot of good passed between us. In all its messy glory, my yoga education was good. Not perfect, but good enough.

I am sympathetic to those with different perspectives based on the time they spent with him. Clearly, many people felt the ethics violations were significant, so some of my views are not going to be useful to them. In cases of abuse especially, a different set of boundaries—internal and external—may be needed for healing.

Recently, the minister of my local church was preaching about how "to bring love and oneness to life" within our daily lives. Her advice centered on "staying in relationship." She described how her family of origin would discuss hot topics, disagree and fight, and yet still were able to remain in relationship as a family around a dinner table. She clarified that "oneness of heart" did not mean not disagreeing; rather, that oneness was lived in the midst of disagreement in the unity of being a family. Then she said, "I must make a caveat here: In cases of abuse, I do not advocate staying in relationship." So, like that. In cases of abuse, ethics violations and the like, many of my (or anyone's) philosophical musings must be applied relative to one's specific situation. None of this work is easy, simple or one-size-fits-all . . . and things often go more wrong than right. We are up to the challenge.

Yoga with God?

One of my psychology mentors once told me that the three most difficult topics to get the average psychotherapy patient to discuss are money, sex and God. I reflect on her words frequently in my work as a yoga teacher. On the mat is potentially where spirituality meets physicality, and many times this meeting calls forth memories and emotions related to past wounds. As yoga has grown in popularity and our class size increases, we no longer offer a strictly counterculture, spiritually-oriented practice "for hippies" . . . as it was in the 70s. The modern yoga class attracts people from a variety of professional, religious, socio-economic and cultural backgrounds.

In America, we might find—or expect to find—a tension between Christianity and yoga, for instance, because so much of the dominant culture in America is Christian. However, the challenges of incorporating spiritual teaching and themes in a public, secular environment such as a yoga class, live outside America as well. For instance, I have taught yoga in a country that was predominantly Muslim, where many of my students left the session for prayer at specified times. And, as much as yoga teachers may worry about offending someone by talking about philosophy, several of my dedicated Christian students have told me they worry they will be judged for their faith in the yoga classroom. Finding a balance where the traditional teachings can be explored within a community that simultaneously values individual expressions of faith is a bit of a moving target.

One obvious solution for these inherent tensions is to leave spiritual teachings out of the yoga classroom. I support that approach for those teachers for whom it feels right. For students who want a "straight asana" class, I suggest that they look until they find a class that meets their needs. There is nothing wrong with calling an asana class what it is, and allowing the work of awareness through breath-based movement and alignment to stand on its own without accompanying philosophical perspectives. And while this straight-asana approach is not my own, I see the value in staying away from the potential hotbed of misunderstandings that can occur within diverse groups when spiritual teachings are introduced without proper context, preparation and time for integration.

For me, however, the value in a postural yoga practice is not only in the way that the poses stretch and strengthen my physical body, but in the way the poses expand my relationship to my inner life. I find that the value in yoga practice lives in the ways philosophy is *brought to life*, in the practical tools for overcoming dysfunctional patterns, and in the ways "God" becomes an internalized experience, as opposed to an outer doctrine or set of rules to follow. Aligning bones, engaging muscles and achieving postures is interesting, captivating and valuable. But I have never found a deeper back bend to be of much use when I was struggling with doubt, despair, addiction, obsession or compulsion. As important as anatomy is, and knowing how to align our bodies is to prevent injury, I have yet to find reliable sources of courage, strength or hope in the outer level of the asana.

Clearly, asana is an exercise for the body. And, the practice includes and initiates a process of moving from the outer layers of body that we can see, taste, touch, hear and smell to increasingly more subtle layers of awareness. Eventually, to the awareness of Awareness itself.

In fact, some yogic texts refer to the "Great It" as "Awareness" or "Consciousness" . . . not to "God"—a useful insight into the nature of this Ultimate Reality.

From this perspective, any awareness we cultivate in a physical practice—from where we place our feet, to how we engage our muscles, to how we position ourselves in a room—and any "awareness of our awareness" that grows within us over time, embeds us in the very fabric of Reality, in Consciousness in the form of our own conscious placement and engagement. Whether we talk about spirituality in class or not, the practice rests in a context of awareness. Participating in the context of awareness consciously increases the efficacy of our efforts and expands our capacity to find greater depth and meaning in and through a physically-oriented endeavor.

That being said, sometimes just hearing those three letters together—G*O*D—can wreak havoc on many people's inner peace. And usually for good reasons. From horrific abuses of power to a culturally-endorsed mood of cynicism and suspicion, the word and notion of "God" is problematic for many people. In my trainings, I often jokingly instruct participants that, "If the three-letter word gives you trouble, make it a four-letter word: LOVE."

The invocation on the following page is a traditional mantra used between teachers and students as they embark upon study together.

It is a prayer that in our togetherness as teachers and students we are:

- protected
- spiritually nourished
- made strong in spirit
- filled with Purpose
- made radiant
- free from hostility and the seeds of enmity for one another
- full of peace.

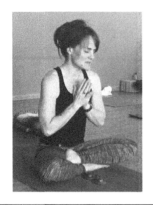

Invocation

om
saha nāvavatu
saha nau bhunaktu
saha vīryaṃ karavāvahai
tejasvinā vadhīta mastu
mā vidviṣāvahai
oṃ śāntiḥ śāntiḥ śāntiḥ

I believe this chant refers to the exoteric (outer and more obvious) level of the teacher–student relationship as well as the more esoteric (interior and subtler) level of the teacher–student relationship. As a yoga teacher, I want these stated qualities to manifest in my classroom as much as possible.

Additionally, I want those same qualities for each of my students internally, so that the recognition and expression of these virtues does not depend on me as the teacher or on being in the classroom. Yoga is a process of education and learning. In yoga, we can learn to use the outer teacher, teachings and practices to draw our innate wisdom, compassion and depth of Spirit forth from within, so that we become a student of our own wisdom and direct experience, as opposed to being dependent on or at the mercy of an outside source. In this way, education empowers not because someone else grants the power, but because students claim the power of their own understanding and authority.

Obviously, good teachers have expertise, knowledge, information and experience to share with their students. A knowledgeable and experienced teacher is a significant aid in any educational endeavor.

However, the teacher's essential job is to create circumstances and learning environments that will encourage their students' innate wisdom to unfold. When the inner wisdom unfolds in the students, they can draw forth from within themselves the qualities they need to cope during troubled times, whether those troubled times are personal, cultural or a combination of both. When yoga is engaged as the inside-out proposition I am describing, the teacher is freed from unrealistic standards of perfection and the student is freed from potentially complicated psychological dynamics such as co-dependency, coercion, transference and projection caused by the inherent power differentials of the teacher-student relationship.

Learning to access, trust and rely upon our inner wisdom is often easier said than done. Like any respectful and enduring relationship, this kind of intimacy with ourselves takes time. And, while the rewards are great, the lessons rarely come cheaply. Recognizing and acknowledging the difficulty and rewards of the learning process can help both teachers and students have compassion for one another, lower unrealistic expectations of the learning process itself, and discover a humble and clear foundation upon which to build.

This chant can serve as a powerful reminder that our life of practice and our relationship with our outer teachers, as well as with our direct experience, need not be cause for self-hatred, self-criticism or enmity in any way. By invoking blessings of protection, spiritual nourishment, strength, purpose, freedom from the seeds of hatred, and peace, this chant offers us a moment to enter into the teacher-student relationship with the intention that the process be as peaceful as possible and aimed at the best possible outcome for all.

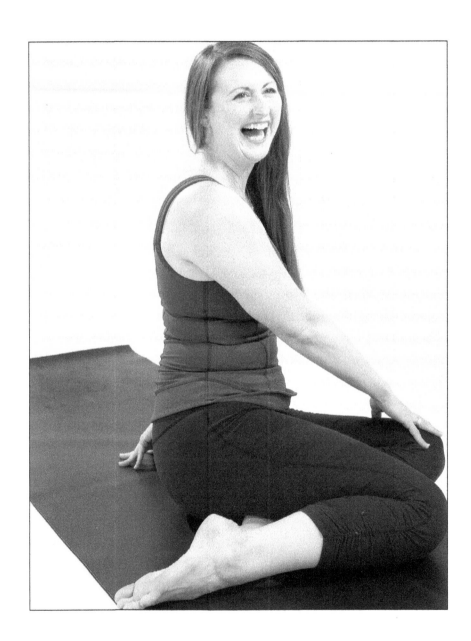

EPILOGUE

RISE UP

In the fall of last year, a visiting Episcopalian bishop came to our church and preached about Lazarus. For those not familiar with this story from the Christian Gospel, Jesus receives a message that Lazarus (brother of Mary and Martha) is ill, and the two sisters are seeking Jesus's help. Jesus's disciples do not want him to go, but that doesn't stop him. By the time he and his followers arrive in Bethany, Lazarus is already dead and buried four days ago. Before they enter the town, Martha meets Jesus and seemingly upbraids him: "If you had been here, my brother would not have died." But he immediately assures her that her brother will rise again.

When Jesus and his group arrive at Lazarus' tomb and remove the stone that covered the entrance, Jesus, after praying to God, calls in a loud voice, "Lazarus, rise up and come forth!" To the astonishment of all, the dead man comes out, his hands and feet still wrapped with strips of linen and a cloth around his face. Then Jesus says to the assembly, "Take off the grave clothes and let him go."

The visiting minister suggested that each of us was each person in this story in some way, and at some time in our lives. Each one of us, like Jesus, is called to help, to heal, to respond to someone's suffering. Each one of us is the disciple warning Jesus not to go, worrying about the dangers of the task we are called to, resistant to the cry we have heard. Each one of us is Martha, accusing and blaming God that he wasn't there to spare us from misfortune.

More significantly, each one of us is Lazarus, bound and blinded by habits of thought, word and deed that keep us locked in a tomb of limitation. And, perhaps most importantly, each one of us can *rise up* and *come forth* through the power of love. Each one of us can be renewed, revived and, dare I say, *resurrected* in love.

Almost five years before her death, my mom had her second stroke. This one came thirteen years after her first stroke, and her recovery from the second one had been difficult for her, for dad and for our family. As her needs increased, we made the choice for both my parents to move together to an assisted living community. While we struggled to make the best choice we could for them at the time, it turned out that this new place was depressing for them both. Our family then decided to relocate them to Colorado so they could live with my husband and me.

Mom didn't talk much after her second stroke; she had slipped into her inner world to a degree that we as a family were unsure if she were experiencing signs of dementia or if she had a more significant level of damage from the stroke than we had previously thought. In the time she lived with us, her strength increased, her interest in life returned and she initiated telling stories, making jokes and laughing at herself and all of us. In more ways than I can list, she, like Lazarus, came back to life.

Caring for both my parents in this way was clearly a good thing for them, and I am grateful to have been a part of this transition period. Our new arrangement was beneficial for me also. In countless small and often seemingly insignificant ways, the change breathed new life into my perspectives, unbound areas of my own self-centeredness and opened my eyes to a wider world of loving. Love called me out of a cave of comfort into an arena of risk that continues to hold its own reward in the process of living into it. I, too, like Lazarus, rose up, came forth and stepped into a new life in love.

The thing about love . . . it has the power to transform, not only those who receive it but those who offer it. Being a part of someone's depression lifting, witnessing someone's sense of humor returning, and providing a place someone can call "home" is deep, meaningful and extraordinary territory to inhabit. Tender, precious, tough and worthwhile.

I think *learning* yoga is difficult. Each one of us steps into the classroom—be it a public class, an online offering, a workshop or a training—with a unique set of circumstances including, but not limited to, our personal history, our current lifestyle, our hopes and dreams, our strengths and weaknesses, our unchecked biases and our privileges and disadvantages. For all of our similarities, we are also different, with variables too numerous to name.

I also think *teaching* yoga is difficult. Teachers vary in education, expertise, charisma, compassion, dedication, maturity, depth and skill. Learning environments range from private sessions to gym classes to public parks to eclectic studios to studios dedicated to a singular approach of study and practice. Some teachers are articulate in their own bodies, but give confusing cues. Some teachers give great cues, but don't know why what they say seems to work. Some teachers are kind but inexperienced. Some are seasoned but impatient. Some are poetic. Some are concrete. Some are practical. Some are mystical. And so on.

And, if you set aside learning styles, teaching styles, personality preferences and limitations galore, the subject matter of yoga still is as vast as the ocean. Each one of us comes to the shores of the subject dressed for gym class, holding a tiny little cup called "our current capacity" and eager to engage a sophisticated, physically- and psychologically-complex endeavor that is often set to music and crammed in between appointments and family obligations. Nonetheless, we do our best to learn.

A DEEPER YOGA

To my continued amazement, for all of the misinformation, confusion and problems that exist, the process *works* for many people. I do not mean it works perfectly or that it never fails. Certainly, enough evidence exists about the abysmal failures of teachers, systems, communities and practitioners; it would be ludicrous to suggest nothing is broken or that nothing needs to be improved. Still, I know I am doing my best to make changes to my teaching that best reflect my current understanding of my past mistakes.

Through it all, I see people *find* each other. Enduring friendships form in these rooms. I see people find themselves and begin the process of making peace with long-forgotten places of pain and previously unknown sources of beauty. I see bodies get stronger and more mobile. I see discernment dawn in simple acts such as modified postures and intelligent questions. I see people choose to spend time, money and attention to explore who they are through the practices of yoga. I see these same people stay with that process through every great joy and tragedy that life can dish out. My friends, students, colleagues and teachers on the path have practiced through births and deaths, marriages and divorces, abortions, miscarriages, murders, abuse, manipulation, disappointments and anything else you can name. And for every triggered trauma, we also have healing, reparative and corrective experiences.

Like for Lazarus, I have seen the practice *rise up* inside each of us when we least expected it: We remember to breathe, we know how to respond to someone we love, we shut up, we speak out, we expand beyond our body of habits in some small way that creates just enough room for a new possibility to emerge. Of course, we fall short also. Obviously, despite our best intentions we make mistakes. We miss the mark. But, there are moments ... moments when we can glimpse that all our yoga was not a "time out" from a busy or stressful life, but was, instead, a training in warriorship, a preparation for service and an exercise in compassion.

146

Rise Up

My spiritual teacher Lee used to say that there were three times in life when we are most available to Divine Influence: When we are praying; when we are laughing; and when we think nothing is going on. I am pretty big into prayer and I am a pretty funny yoga teacher, but I have to say that I think most of my life of practice and teaching falls into the third domain he mentioned. I rarely think that anything very meaningful is happening in my effort to do *trikonasana* or to push up to *urdhva dhanurasana*. I do not roll out my mat most days with lofty aims or high intentions. I mostly practice with an "another day, another down dog" kind of mentality, much in the same way I brush my teeth.

And yet.

And yet.

And yet, something seems to have been built. And I see it in my students also. I have the good fortune to have been teaching long enough for some students to have been practicing with me for over twenty years. I have come to see that learning, practicing, teaching and living are a long-term relationship and not a one-night stand. And like any long-term relationship, there are good times and bad, tough moments as well as tender ones.

Living authentically through these unavoidable tough and tender times is what a deeper yoga is all about. In the face of injustice, suffering and difficulty, a deeper yoga that moves us beyond image and conditioning to the depths of the Self within is a lifeline to sanity, sanctity and hope. We live in difficult times, when forces seem to be stacked in favor of despair, cynicism and nihilism. In the face of such odds, it is easy to overlook small acts of courage and affirmation and to discount our individual contributions, be those contributions a well-taught yoga class, making dinner or finding time for true self-care. Whatever positive action you can take, I urge you to stay in the game and to invest in whatever expression of love, hope and faith that you can muster today.

And in the words of one of my teachers, "Keep practicing. It makes all the difference."

RESOURCES

Yoga and Body Image

The Yoga and Body Image Coalition

The Yoga and Body Image Coalition is committed to body love by developing, promoting and supporting yoga that is accessible, body positive and reflects the full range of human diversity. Our mission not only advocates yoga as an essential tool in personal transformation, from the inside out, but also includes a critical social justice component by challenging industry leaders and media creators to expand their vision of what a yogi looks like.
www.ybicoalition.com

Hunger, Hope + Healing
Sarahajoy Marsh

Sarahjoy Marsh offers her personal and professional experience to help you use yoga to reclaim your relationship to your body and food. With important topics such as understanding compulsion, overcoming anxiety, and moving from love not shame, Sarah's down-to-earth approach is practical and inspiring.
www.sarahjoyyoga.com/hungerhopeandhealing.html

Curvy Yoga

Anna Guest Jelly believes that yoga and body acceptance come together through practice. Together, they create an experience she calls Curvy Yoga Practice—a highly individualized process for you to bring both yoga and body acceptance into your life in regular, doable ways.
www.curvyyoga.com

Diane Bondy Yoga

Dianne Bondy is a celebrated yoga teacher, social justice activist and leading voice of the *Yoga For All* movement. Her inclusive view of yoga asana and philosophy inspires and empowers thousands of followers around the world, regardless of their shape, size, ethnicity, or level of ability. Dianne contributes to *Yoga International, Yoga Journal, Do You Yoga*, and *Elephant Journal*. She is featured and profiled in International media outlets: The Guardian, Huffington Post, Cosmopolitan, and more. She is a spokesperson for diversity in yoga and yoga for larger bodies, as seen in her work with Pennington's, Gaiam, and the Yoga & Body Image Coalition. Her work is published in the books: *Yoga and Body Image*, and *Yes Yoga Has Curves*.

www.dianebondyyoga.com

Meditation and Philosophy Studies

Luminous Soul Studies

The Luminous Soul Method is a unique system that guides students through nine pillars. Each pillar has key principles and practical tools that unlock your happiness and joyful living within your modern life. As you grow in the Luminous Soul Method, you learn the nine pillars. The more you understand a pillar the more you build what Manorama, the founder, calls "essential core strengths," which give you confidence in your yogic practice and ease in your life. In the Luminous Soul Method, Manorama guides you in working with elements such as ancient Sanskrit texts, Luminous Soul weekly exercises and wisdom discussions, and opens up what she calls "archetypal patterns." As you work with her Luminous Soul Method pillars, you move from a life of *stuck and unrealized*, to a life of *purpose, strength and confidence*. And you learn how to consciously bridge your everyday experiences with the meaningful and spiritual.

www.sanskritstudies.org

Blue Throat Yoga

Based on the daily practice of Neelakantha Meditation, you are invited to return home into your own heart, settling deeply inside to access the natural bliss, ease and beauty of life itself. Neelakantha Meditation comes from the ancient Tantric teachings of Svatantra, the true freedom of

Consciousness, and is offered by Master Teacher, Dr. Paul Muller-Ortega, as well as by the Authorized Teachers of Neelakantha Meditation located in the U.S. and abroad, in a perfectly contemporary form that supports and uplifts "householder" or daily life for everyone.
www.bluethroatyoga.com

Carlos Pomeda

Originally from Madrid, Spain, Carlos has been steeped in all aspects of the yoga tradition during more than forty years of practice and study. He spent eighteen of those years as a monk of the Saraswati order, under the name Swami Gitananda, including nine years of traditional training and practice in India. As a teacher, Carlos is renowned for the breadth of his knowledge and the clarity with which he conveys it. His great love of the Indian yoga traditions, his insight, his humor and his deep connection with his audiences give him the ability to transmit the deepest scriptural teachings in a way that is clear, meaningful and applicable.
www.pomeda.com

Sally Kempton

Sally Kempton is one of today's most authentic spiritual teachers. She teaches devotional contemplative tantra—an approach to practice that creates a fusion of knowing and loving. Known for her ability to transmit inner experience through transformative practices and contemplation, Sally has been practicing and teaching for forty years. She now offers heart-to-heart transmission in meditation and life practice through her Awakened Heart Tantra workshops, teleclasses, retreats, and trainings in applied spiritual philosophy. Her workshops and teleconference courses integrate the wisdom of traditional yoga tantra with the insights of contemporary evolutionary spirituality and cutting-edge psychology.
www.sallykempton.com

Asana Studies with Christina Sell

To find out more about how to study in person or online with Christina Sell, please visit her website at www.livethelightofyoga.com.

INDEX

conditioning, 10, 24, 27, 78, 117, 147
  cultural, 64
consciousness, 21, 48, 87, 94, 106, 110
  Absolute, 64, 139
  expanded, 40, 78, 83
consistency, 103, 104
context, 28, 35, 91, 97, 100, 101, 115, 117, 124, 138
  of awareness, 139
  and curiosity, 110
  and practice, 108, 120
  and prajna, 106
conventional(ly), 32, 35, 78, 86
  society, 7, 8, 43, 81
curiosity, 68, 100, 101, 110
Curvy Yoga, 148

D
Day-Lewis, C., 100
devotion, 9, 58, 68, 75, 92, 117
dieting, 4, 54
direct experience, xx, 3, 23, 25, 58, 115, 140, 141
  of love, 13, 94
dukha (duhkhabhaag), 86
dysmorphia, 21, 56

E
eating disorder, x, 21, 40, 54, 57, 58
education(al), 27, 64, 115-118, 133
  as a process, 140
  and the intellect, 122
effect(s), 21, 64
  cumulative, 3, 84
efforts, 13, 29, 103-105, 108
  effects of, 20, 37, 44, 64, 139
  sustained, xvii, xix, 24
ektara, xix
Elliot, Lang, 80
energy, 15, 20, 39, 62, 77, 81, 104
  depleting, 35

directing, 102
emotional, 66
field of, 10, 78, 129
group, 124
outgoing, 19
positive, 45
stuck, 99
entrainment, 82, 83
essence
  inner, 25, 81
  of practice, ii
  of love, xx
  spiritual, 23
essential
  nature, 19, 86
  Self, 37
exercise, xvi, 3, 5, 70
  compulsive, xvii, 4, 56

F
faith, 12, 92, 102, 103, 107, 138, 147
fear, 10, 12, 19, 33, 34, 43, 55, 118, 126
  paying attention to, 47, 70
feeling(s), 22-24, 55, 65-68, 95, 118
  observing, 46, 47, 70, 105
food, xiv-xvi, 19, 53, 57-59, 62, 64-66, 69, 148. *See also* addiction
  types of, 61

G
Gitananda, Swami, 150
Goldberg, Natalie, 100
grief, 67, 118
group setting, 27, 28
guru, 82-84

H
Haunted Heart: The Life and Times of Stephen King, The (Rogak), 104
healing, 6, 25, 45, 87, 88, 133, 136, 146
  perfectionism, 39, 40

Index

power of, xvii, 5, 27
heart, 4, 11, 19, 36, 94, 106, 119, 126, 137,149
  opening, 118
  self-compassion, 49
  spiritual, 25, 71
  writing and the, 14
hero's journey, 19
hot studio, 116
hunger, 54, 61
  emotional, 65, 66, 68, 69
  intellectual, 63
  physical, 62, 69
  spiritual, 68
Hunger, Hope + Healing, 148

I

identification(s), 9, 57, 78, 79, 105, 106
information stage, 120-122
injuries, 116, 134
injury, xvii, xx, 47, 138
innate wisdom, 121, 140, 141
inspiration, 21, 27, 41, 82, 115, 117-119, 123, 124, 130
instinct(s), 11, 65, 70, 117, 118
integration, 13, 41, 86, 115, 117, 127, 128, 130, 138
integrity, 9, 11, 20
intellect, 63, 65, 110, 122, 123
interdependence, 6, 80
interpersonal skills, 120
intimacy, 28, 48, 67, 127, 131, 141

J

Jelly, Anna Guest, 148
Jesus, 102, 143

K

Kempton, Sally, 150

L

Lazarus, 143-146
life
  inner, 20, 47, 55, 57, 109, 138
  outer, 19, 20, 84
"light of the soul," 19
limit(s), 6, 31, 45, 48, 118, 122, 125,
love, xv, xvii, xix, xx, 17, 32-38, 49, 75, 83, 87-95, 144, 145
  conditional, 40
  field of, 13, 38, 46, 94
  flow of, 87
  See also self-love
Lozowick, Lee, xviii, 53, 90, 97, 156
Luminous Soul Studies, 149

M

Manorama, 149
mantra, 34, 40, 89, 108, 139
Marsh, Sarahajoy, 148
Matthew 17:20, 103
meditation, 39, 47, 84, 103, 106, 109, 116, 129, 149
  Loving Kindness, 88
Muller-Ortega, Dr. Paul, 150

N

nature, 80-82, 110, 134
Neelakantha Meditation, 149, 150
Neff, Kristin, 44
non-rational, 65, 110

O

obsessive, 24, 34, 55, 57, 62
Oliver, Mary, 82
oppression, 22, 43, 118
orientation, 65, 109
  external, 9
  inner, 23, 38

P

Patanjali, 102, 106
pay(ing) attention, 20, 21, 47, 48, 58, 69,
perfection
    -ism, 32, 35, 37, 39, 40, 45, 58, 101
    -istic, 35, 39, 40, 44, 108, 117
physical expression, 63, 134
Poetic Image, The (Day-Lewis), 100
Pomeda, Carlos, 150
poses, 20, 23, 35, 44, 48, 49, 78, 128, 138. *See also* asana
    timed, 124
postural practice, xvii, 35, 46, 138
practice, xv, xvii, xix, 9, 13, 36, 45-49, 69, 81, 84, 104
    inspiration for, 118, 119
    personal, xviii, 3-6, 23, 26-28, 92, 93, 116, 129, 146
    process of, 65, 102, 105, 108, 122, 121, 125, 126
    spiritual, 6, 12, 17, 25, 38, 44, 53, 65, 70, 89, 90, 137
    theory of, 64, 120, 123, 124
    writing, 14, 95, 103, 123
    yoga, 8, 10, 16, 33-35, 39, 40, 75, 77, 115, 134, 138
prajna, 102, 106
prana, 77
pranayama, 28, 38, 40, 48, 89, 108
prayer, 68, 86, 87, 139
psyche, 110
psychological, 32, 37, 40, 44, 47, 88, 92
    dynamics, 122, 141
    patterns, 117, 134
purge, 54, 55
purna, 31

R

Reality, xviii, 8, 53, 54, 139
recovery
    from addiction, 54-56, 62, 78, 120
    12-step program, xiv, 44, 93
reference point(s), 3, 17, 32, 38, 71, 75, 81, 125
    expanded, 6, 11, 77, 84, 85
    external, 9, 45
    inner, 10, 83, 94
regularity, 103, 104
rishis, 128
Rogak, Lisa, 104

S

sages, 20, 128
salvation, 22, 46
samadhi, 102, 105-107
sanctuary, 115, 121, 122
self
    -acceptance, 37, 97, 102
    -compassion, xviii, 43-46, 48, 49
    -criticism, xvii, 13, 21, 37, 48, 71, 103, 141
    -esteem, 5, 22
      negative, xvii
    -hatred, 24, 27, 37, 53, 141
    -love, xvii, 11, 36, 43, 46, 48, 57
    -regard, 46
    -talk, 45
      negative, 5, 24
    -understanding, 3, 15, 23, 75, 77, 98, 102
Sell, Christina, 5, 17, 32, 41, 131, 150
separation, 5, 22
service, xix, 58, 146
shame, 11, 25, 27, 48, 49, 55, 65, 75, 76, 78, 98, 148
    as suffering, 46
    -based, 24
    body, 56

Index

ABOUT THE AUTHOR

CHRISTINA SELL has been practicing asana since 1991 and teaching since 1998. She believes that yoga practice can help anyone access their inner wisdom and authentic spirituality, and clarify their highest personal expression.

Christina has a BA in Counseling and an MA in Integrative Education. She maintains an active teaching schedule presenting seminars locally, nationally and internationally. A devoted student of Western Baul master, Lee Lozowick, she credits his Influence as the spiritual inspiration behind her life and work.

Christina resides in Buena Vista, Colorado with her husband, her aging father, her dog, and two very affectionate kitty cats. She enjoys practicing yoga, writing, reading, cooking, hiking, mountain biking, and snowboarding. She is the author of: *Yoga from the Inside Out* and *My Body Is a Temple* (both from Hohm Press).

CONTACT: For more information about her and her work, please visit her website www.livethelightofyoga.com

ABOUT HOHM PRESS

HOHM PRESS is committed to publishing books that provide readers with alternatives to the materialistic values of the current culture, and promote self-awareness, the recognition of interdependence, and compassion. Our subject areas include parenting, transpersonal psychology, religious studies, women's studies, the arts and poetry.

CONTACT INFORMATION: Hohm Press, PO Box 4410, Chino Valley, Arizona, 86323; USA; 800-381-2700, or 928-636-3331; email: publisher@hohmpress.com

Visit our website at www.hohmpress.com